Younger Next Year*

THE Exercise Program

The Companion to the
New York Times Bestseller

Chris Crowley &
Henry S. Lodge, M.D.

With a Whole-Body Exercise Regimen
by Bill Fabrocini, P.T.

WORKMAN PUBLISHING • NEW YORK

Most of this book was previously published in 2004 in *Younger Next Year* and in 2012 in
Thinner This Year.

Library of Congress Cataloging-in-Publication Data is available.

ISBN: 978-0-7611-8612-0

Cover and layout design by Ariana Abud
Technical illustrations by James Williamson

Photo Credits: fotolia: Mostafa Fawzy—pp. 15, 17, 25, 32, 35, 39, 65, 67, 69, 77, 116; Susan
Montgomery—p. 41; rashadashurov—p. 40; Sam—p. 110; tulpahn—p. 36.

Workman books are available at special discounts when purchased in bulk for premiums
and sales promotions as well as for fund-raising or educational use. Special editions or book
excerpts can also be created to specification. For details, contact the Special Sales Director at
the address below or send an email to specialmarkets@workman.com.

Workman Publishing Co., Inc.
225 Varick St.
New York, NY 10014
workman.com
youngernextyear.com

WORKMAN is a registered trademark of Workman Publishing Co., Inc.

Printed in China
First printing January 2016

10 9 8 7 6 5 4 3 2 1

The program of exercise in *Younger Next Year: The Exercise Program* is safe and
scientifically structured. Nevertheless, consult your doctor before beginning this or any
exercise program—particularly if you have ever had a heart attack or been diagnosed with
cardiovascular or coronary heart disease; have frequent chest pains or often feel faint or dizzy
upon physical exertion; have high blood pressure or high cholesterol levels, diabetes, or liver
or kidney disease; are female and more than three months pregnant or less than three months
postpartum; or are under eighteen years of age. In addition, ask your doctor's advice if you
have muscle, joint, or bone problems that might be aggravated by exercise. And for Pete's
sake, if you don't feel well or if something hurts, stop.

To Bill Fabrocini,
who teaches us all so much.
—C. C.

This book is dedicated to my patients,
from whom I have learned so much;
and to my family, especially Laura,
my inspiration and touchstone in so many ways;
and to Madeleine and Samantha,
my wellsprings of joy.
—H.S.L.

Contents

Endurance Aerobics • Intervals • Four Interval
Days • Spin Class • A Rowing Machine or Scull
Interval Day • How High to Take Your Heart Rate
During Intervals • Half-Baked Intervals

Introduction

Why another exercise book, and why this book specifically? Because your life should be better. Much better. And recent science has revolutionized our understanding of how exercise can reshape your body, your brain, and your life. We explained the why and the how of exercise in our previous *Younger Next Year* books, and Chris's book, *Thinner This Year*.

Chris Crowley is my patient, dear friend, and partner in writing these books. More important, he is the living, breathing, exuberant voice of vibrant aging in America. Chris is out there living all of our dreams, and his whole purpose in life is to pull you into the dream with him.

In this book, we take the best information from *Younger Next Year* and the innovative exercise programs from *Thinner This Year* to give you a road map to your best life. And what a life it can be!

In the decade since we wrote the *Younger* books, new scientific research has only underscored our fundamental message about exercise. A serious exercise program will keep you healthier, more engaged, and living younger for the rest of your life. Physical fitness reverses most of the inflammation of modern life—heart disease, stroke, diabetes, most of arthritis—all of the things that we associate with normal American aging. You become a much better version of yourself, at any age, and you become functionally younger. Not by months, or years, but by decades. A seventy-year-old man or woman who follows our program will have the aerobic capacity of a healthy forty-five-year-old. You really can live twenty-five years younger than your driver's license says almost all the way through your life.

And your brain will get younger, too. Newer research has shown that there are enormous cognitive benefits of exercise. The data and individual biology vary, but when you are fit, you are 10 percent more cognitively efficient than when you are sedentary. Simply put, your brain does more, and it does it better. Interestingly, sleep does the same thing. So the fit, rested version of you is about 20 percent smarter than the tired, out-of-shape you. And that's in addition to the health and longevity benefits of exercise. That's why we think your best life is still waiting for you. With this book in your hands and sweating.

It's often said, and accurately, that your brain is the most complex, sophisticated object in the known universe—100 billion neurons, each with up to 10,000 connections to other neurons—dwarfing the Internet in information flow and challenging scientists to develop entirely new branches of mathematics to try to understand it. The federal government recently funded the ten-year BRAIN Initiative to examine the connections and cross talk among all the areas of the brain because that's where the vast majority of brain processing takes place. This new frontier of brain science is important because our brains work by synthesizing vast amounts of data from many sources. As you read this, your brain is primarily processing the visual information of the text. But it's also keenly aware of your emotions, physical surroundings, internal chemistry, and your body's position in space. It's the fusion of these disparate inputs that creates our consciousness and consciousness rests on a base of physical information.

So what do you do to turn on this most complex object in the universe? Watch TV on the sofa? Putz around online? No. Your brain grows best when it is given challenges that involve many areas at once. And there are only three great challenges that are hard enough to keep the brain healthy and growing. True emotional engagement with others, cognitive and social engagement with tasks that matter, and exercise. Motion. Moving your body through space is unbelievably complicated. We take it for granted, but even simple movement requires the entire brain to coordinate body parts. Movement is at the heart of evolution, it's key for improving our cognitive and emotional brains.

Let's look at how exercise transforms your brain for the long haul. One study showed a 40 percent reduction in the risk of Alzheimer's in people who do some kind of aerobic activity regularly. Other studies, using very careful measurements of brain size on MRI scans, showed that people who exercise for three months grow new brain. And the new brain is not just in the motion areas, where you would expect it, but also in the frontal cortex, the area of the brain that controls executive function (complex thoughts, rational calculations, decision making, etc.).

Just as impressively, you change the brain chemistry of your emotions as well. It has now been shown that exercise is as effective as medication in treating both anxiety and depression. Exercise releases a powerful brain chemistry that in turn creates the energy, optimism, and mood elevation you need in order to engage with life at your best. This is important for many reasons, not least because American longevity is increasing at a stunning rate. Statistically, you are likely to live a long time. The big question in this book is how well will you live that life?

There is a lot of debate over *why* we are living longer. Modern medicine gets some credit. Cutting the smoking rate in half in the last fifty years has been a major contributor, but whatever is driving this increase in longevity, there is no doubt that it is happening, and in a big way. American life expectancy has been increasing by about four hours a day since the 1970s (that means that every day you live beyond age sixty-five, you add four hours to your life expectancy). Financial planners now tell healthy couples in their sixties to plan on at least one of them living to ninety-five. Even this might be conservative.

Recently I gave a talk about the future of aging, and it was an opportunity for me to pick some very smart brains at Columbia University, which is an international leader in this area. No one knows what's going to happen, but here's my take: For the next decade, the increase will continue at around the current rate. In ten to twenty years, we will probably figure out more effective ways to individualize medical care through genomic medicine (using your individual genetics to tailor diagnosis and treatment specifically for you *and* the genetics of your infection or cancer). In the twenty- to thirty-year range we might (*might*) be able to alter the fundamental genetics of human longevity. We can already extend the life span of worms tenfold, and add a third to the lives of mice through simple genetic manipulation, so real progress in this area is likely. How much is open to debate, as are a host of ethical and social concerns, but those have never stopped progress.

So congratulations! We got longevity, whether we wanted it or not. Now, what are we going to do with it? The problem with the new longevity is that so many Americans outlive the quality component of their lives by years, and even decades. Some of this is unavoidable, but because 70 percent of our illness and injury is lifestyle related, most of the misery and limitations of aging are self-imposed—the natural outcome of the biology of sedentary living. Some of it is because our expectations are mired in an outdated cultural model: We think aging is going to be grim, and our actions ensure that the prophecy is fulfilled.

If you ask people about growing old, they will give you the standard, gloomy answer, which is some variation of "aging is hard, full of aches, pains, and loss." Loss of function, loss of friends, loss of purpose—all summed up by the adage "aging is not for sissies." Not that those things aren't real, and hard parts of aging, but they are more than offset by surprising positive aspects. The actual views about aging from the front lines are far better than you think and will change your perspective on the last third of life. If, instead of generic questions, you ask what a person's actual experience is as he or she grows older, you get a very different answer from the old cultural narrative. Researchers have studied aging in cultures around the world, and the positive results are remarkably consistent across continents and societies.

It turns out that we continue to grow as people throughout our lives, and that the years from our fifties onward are times of enormous personal growth, change, and reinvention. Research into aging has undergone a marked shift in the last decade, with the recognition of the tremendous potential for happy and productive lives for many, if not most, of us through our seventies, into our eighties, and in some cases into our nineties. There are few long-term studies of people over the course of their lives, but one is the Harvard Grant Study of Aging, which follows a group of Harvard college students from the late 1930s and 1940s. The different trajectories of the lives of these men, now in their eighties and nineties, show that they continued to grow and evolve, finding new passions, meeting new challenges, and carving out new definitions of self, community, and relationships throughout their lives. (There are some similar studies for women, but they aren't as long-term. Nonetheless, the data tell the same story.) There is no static plateau, where you have finished growing and stay the same for the rest of your life. You continue to *live*. And for most people studied, it continues to be exciting and meaningful, even happy.

Surprisingly, self-reported life satisfaction/happiness goes down from your midtwenties through your early fifties, probably representing the stress of the years of raising children, establishing one's career, dealing with the financial strain of mortgages, tuition, etc. These are also years when you are struggling to figure out who you are as an adult, carving your place in the world, having your successes and your failures, and ultimately becoming comfortable with what you have, or have not, achieved. By your midfifties, this phase of life—when you are completing the major tasks of career and family—is over, and you are looking forward to retirement, which seems like the ultimate negative definition of self. ("I'm retired" defines you as who you *used* to be but says nothing about who you *are* and, more important, offers no excitement about who you *are going to be*.) So you would expect the data to show less happiness in the later years.

It turns out that happiness goes *up* from your midfifties onward, not down. And the curve continues upward at a steep rate at least into your early eighties, which is as far as studies have measured. When you look at the happiness graph that follows, it looks like a lopsided smile, with the biggest grin on the older side of the curve.

Good news! It can be life-changing for people to learn that the last third is every bit as dynamic and full of possibility as the first two-thirds and in some ways more so, because you are freed of many of the emotional burdens you carried when younger.

So what can go wrong with this happy picture? Well, bad luck

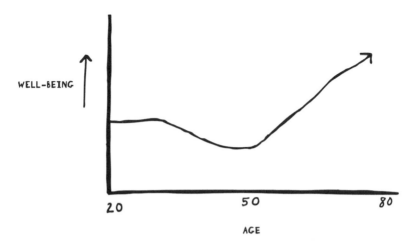

WELL-BEING

20   50   80

AGE

in terms of devastating illness or loss, but aside from that, if it is not going well it may be because you passively let aging happen to you. For most of us, the downward slide is a choice. As I said earlier, 70 percent of the illnesses we are prone to are lifestyle related, and you can take a lot of them off the table, including, surprisingly, a lot of Alzheimer's, most of the heart attacks and strokes, almost all of the type 2 diabetes, and the majority of arthritis and obesity. Getting weak and out of shape (scientists now call it the "frailty of the elderly") is different from getting sick; it is not a disease, it simply prevents you from living anything but a diminished life. It does lead to illness and infections because your immune system gets weak along with you, but the biggest issue, for our purposes, is the marked reduction in your quality of life. Couple this with the prospects of longevity, and you have a dismal picture of long, grim aging. The key point from *Younger Next Year*, and even more true today, is that *this is not really aging*. It's *decay*. And *it is optional. It's a choice you make* by how you live. You can choose to grow instead, and have a vibrant, meaningful life almost all the way through. Sadly, decay has become the norm for the majority of

Americans. It can now start in our forties, or even earlier, in the near-criminal lifestyle abuse we impose on our children. If you look at the arteries of an obese child under a microscope, they look exactly like the arteries of a forty-five-year-old. That is the power of decay! But there are a substantial and growing minority who have embraced the challenge and opportunity of aging and are determined to rewrite the rule book.

As you now know, the key to changing those decay signals back to growth is consistent, daily exercise. Exercise is the master signal for growth because it is the language of the physical brain, which runs our bodies and our metabolism. And there's surprising new information on that front as well. Exercise literally changes the gene expression in the muscles, joints, and cells throughout the body. You get to rewrite your genetic code on a daily basis and become far younger than we ever imagined was possible. The best way to illustrate this is by looking at peak athletic performance. You and Chris and I will never be peak athletes, but it's a place where we can measure achievement and compare today's older athletes with past generations, so it shines a light on our potential as well. There are new data that high-end fitness can dramatically slow the muscle loss of aging and the reduction in maximum heart rate. The new approaches to strength, fitness, and conditioning that we show you in this book will introduce you to a whole new, optimistic landscape for aging.

You can see the impact of this sort of training in world-class competitive athletes who are pushing the age-related boundaries of their sport. The clearest example may be Dara Torres, who won an Olympic silver medal in her forties in swimming—a discipline where you used to be washed up by the end of your twenties. But she is by no means alone. People are demolishing our expectations for age-related performance all over the place. A friend of Chris's and mine put together a team of four guys over age seventy to do the Race Across America (RAAM) on bicycles. It's a kind of relay race from the Pacific to the Atlantic, where one of the four guys is always on a bike. They did it in six days and thirteen hours, not only shattering the record for seventy-year-olds, but beating the record for sixty-year-olds as well. The record for young men is five days, so they were a hair off the best pace, but for a bunch of guys in their seventies? It's simply amazing.

And you are invited to play. This stuff is inspiring, and if you want to have some inspirational reading, the RAAM book is called *More Than a Race*, and Torres's book is *Age Is Just a Number*. Your potential for your life should inspire *you*—to reach for big goals, to be sure to work up a sweat in the process, and to enjoy it!

As a doctor I find myself talking to patients over and over again about the value of exercise in treating or ameliorating the impact of one or another disease or disability: fractures and osteoporosis, diabetes and stroke. But we also need to remember the fundamental necessity and beauty of exercise. We live in these very confined bodies, now. Our bodies sit, almost all day long, at a desk, behind the steering wheel, etc., and if they move, they move in these very constrained, repetitive ways. We've forgotten how joyful it is to truly move, or what a big deal *play* used to be.When you look at children as they flow through their day, there is a physical joy to movement that is missing from our lives. Past the age of fifty nobody thinks about playing. If we do, it's getting down on the floor to play with kids for a few minutes, and then being too stiff to stand up.

Follow the program that Chris and experts in sports physiology training and body mechanics, Bill Fabrocini and Riggs Klika, have designed for you, and you can regain an amazing amount of playfulness, strength, coordination, balance, fitness, and joy of movement. All at a time in life when people have basically written that off forever. But that's wrong. Our bodies are waiting to be rebuilt in these ways. The energy that comes with a fit body—the cognitive energy, the emotional energy, the optimism—is a powerful surge of goodness in your life as you navigate these years.

The strength exercises in this book are cutting edge. They go beyond the old "pumping iron" approach and introduce you to a world of whole-body movements that train your muscles to work in harmony as you move through space, and let you explore your full physical envelope. Strength training not only reduces the risk of fall and fracture but also gives you back your physical vitality—striding through the world with physical confidence, climbing steps with power and ease, rediscovering agility—joys most Americans thought were lost in the rearview mirror. Fitness training complements this by introducing intensity as a way of supercharging your workout, bringing you to new levels of aerobic endurance and capacity. This book will give you a range of options, from good to great, depending on what you want your life to be and the investment you want to make. Follow the program to get good, and your life will be remarkably good. Follow it to get great, and you will find that for us, great really does mean great.

Now you own the cutting-edge science that will let you change your chemistry, change your body, change your brain, and give you the drive, energy, and sense of purpose to live *your* life on *your* terms for decades to come.

—Henry S. Lodge, M.D., FACP
Robert Burch Family Professor of Medicine,
Columbia University Medical Center

CHAPTER ONE

Why Exercise Matters So Very Much

give talks all over the country these days about exercise and the revolution in aging, the revolution in behavior. It's the most interesting and important thing I do, and I love it. So do the audiences, most of the time. But there is apt to be an uneasy lull, a bit of a dead spot early on, when I tell them that the single most important thing they are going to learn in the next hour—or the next *decade*, come to that—is that it makes a ton of sense for each of them to exercise six days a week for the rest of their lives.

What? You can almost feel their butts shifting in the seats. *"Oh Lord! Who is this guy and why am I here?"* You see their eyes roll up into their skulls as they silently tell themselves, "The chances of my working out six days a week, now or ever, are precisely *zero! Good grief!*"

I spend much of the next hour trying to persuade them that what they just heard is absolutely true. And that, if they buy into it, they will change their lives in wonderful and astonishing ways. Indeed, steady exercise is so critical, and the upside of doing it is so fantastic that the only crazy thing would be *not* doing it. It is at the heart of the revolution in aging.

Harry (that's Henry S. Lodge, M.D., my close friend, my doctor, and the brilliant coauthor of *Younger Next Year*) and I are going to spend a little time here doing the same thing, persuading you *why* a serious program of steady exercise is one of the most important things you can do. Harry will appear in "The Doctor Is In" features throughout the book to tell you about the compelling science behind the program. And we both spell out the jaw-dropping consequences—and the pleasures—of having exercise in your life. Heady stuff, believe me.

But then we shift into the real business of the book . . . the nitty-gritty. We tell you exactly what kind of exercise to do and how to do it. This is the book that Harry's patients, my audiences, and a great many readers of *Younger Next Year* have been asking for—a simple exercise program that will get them through the first months of working out and be solid and detailed enough to serve as *the* reference book for the rest of their lives. For that we rely a lot on two terrific professionals who helped me with the exercise part of the book *Thinner This Year*: Bill Fabrocini, physical therapist, the smartest and best strength trainer I've ever met, and Riggs Klika, Ph.D., a serious student (and now teacher) of the science of aerobic exercise. (More about them in "About the Authors.") Their material is state-of-the-art stuff, believe me.

Our goal is to make this the most important how-to book in your life. A detailed, hands-on guide to the *right way* to exercise. The right way to maximize the impact, to avoid getting hurt, and to enjoy it. It'll be the little book you open at home in the morning, to check on Bill Fabrocini's warm-up program. Or take to the gym to guide you through Bill's cutting-edge strength-training regimen. Or peek at before you throw your leg over your bike or go for a run. We hope you will wear it out, turning backward and forward to refresh yourself. Take it with you everywhere. Why? Because this stuff is so important . . . that's why.

This book is Harry's and my compilation and enhancement of the exercise portions of the *Younger Next Year* books and *Thinner This Year*, which I wrote with Tufts University professor of nutrition and muscle physiology Jen Sacheck, Ph.D. But here the topic is all exercise, which we believe to be the most important part of the revolution in aging. We are tickled to have a handy, single-volume guide that will tell you pretty much everything you need to know about it.

When Do We Begin?

For some reason, an awful lot of our readers are type A lunatics (just like at least one of the authors). And Harry and I both worry that you may get impatient and want to skip ahead to the actual exercises and, for God's sake, *begin*! We get that, but it reflects a deep misunderstanding of what this little book is all about and how it works. The essence of the book is not the exercises, as important as they are. The essence of the book is the long prose buildup that tells you *why* the exercises are important . . . *why* it matters to do them in a certain way. *Why* they work the way they do. *That* is what you will remember. That is what will change your life. *That* is why this may be the most important how-to book you'll ever read. Slow down . . . we're here.

"Come the Revolution . . ."

One of the joys of the last decade for me was that I got to have two year-long tutorials from two of the smartest people I know, Harry Lodge and Jen Sacheck. I was learning about a revolution in aging, a revolution in behavior that will eventually change all of our lives. "Come the revolution," as they used to say. . . . Come the revolution, you will be able to *put off most of aging until almost the end of life*. You will have radically more energy, optimism, effectiveness, be *younger* in all the important ways. *That* is a revolution worth learning about and worth working for. And the heart of it is building yourself a solid exercise program.

I am your basic Wall Street trial lawyer. Not a complete idiot, you know, but a dope about science and medicine. The beauty of the intense tutorial process was that Harry and Jen had to simplify the science behind the revolution enough so that I could understand it—and help pass it on to you. Which is basically what a good trial lawyer does for a living: learns a ton of super-complex material and then passes the *gist of it* on to smart but very busy judges (that's you) who do not have time to go into it all themselves. Quite a privilege for me, I'll tell you, and absolutely fascinating.

The Signaling System

The single most fascinating thing I learned about, during that long stretch of intense (and often difficult) learning, was the body's astonishing signaling system. It turns out that some of the greatest scientific discoveries in recent times involve billions and

⚕ *THE DOCTOR IS IN:* The New Science of Aging

So let's go backstage for a moment to look at the amazing new biology that has transformed our thinking about aging. Biologists now believe that most cells in your body are designed to fall apart after relatively short life spans. The net result is that you are actively destroying large parts of your body all the time. On purpose. To make room for new growth. For example, the muscle cells in your thigh are replaced every four months; you have armies of special cells whose job is to dissolve your bones so other cells can build them up again.

The trick is to grow more than you throw out. This is where exercise comes in. It turns out that your muscles control the chemistry of growth throughout your body. The nerve impulse to contract a muscle also sends a tiny signal to build it up, creating a moment-to-moment chemical balance between growth and decay within the muscle.

So here's the connection: When you exercise fairly hard, you stress your muscles, and you actually injure them slightly. When cells sense the damage from exercise, they automatically release chemicals to start the inflammation. The chemicals that control inflammation are called cytokines; hundreds of them are at work in your body, regulating growth and decay down to the microscopic level. For the purposes of this book, however, imagine that there are only two cytokines—we'll call them cytokine-6 and cytokine-10, or C-6 and C-10, for short. C-6 is the master chemical for inflammation (decay), and C-10 is the master chemical for repair and growth. C-6 is produced in both the muscle cells and the bloodstream in response to exercise, and C-10 is produced in response to C-6. These chemicals leak into the bloodstream, which draws white blood cells (the wrecking crew) to the injured area. This demolition triggers the repair, or growth, process. In other words: *Exercise turns on inflammation, which automatically turns on repair.* So exercise is the master signaler, the agent that sets hundreds of chemical cascades in motion each time you get on the treadmill or take a spin on your bike and start to sweat. Amazing.

billions of signals racing around to every cell in the body, all day long. The system is amazingly subtle and complex; think for a second about the millions of minisignals to the muscles every instant, just to enable us to stand upright . . . to say *nothing* of scratching our noses. Or skiing the double-black diamonds. But curiously, the signals are pretty simple. It's always one of two things: Grow or atrophy. Grow or decay. That's the message to the cells all day long, throughout our lives.

The dance of life, inside our bodies, as in our species, is a dance of growth and decay. This little manual about exercise is in fact nothing less than a dancing lesson . . . to teach you how to *lead* in the dance of life. Sound like a big deal? It should, because it is.

When we are young, the default signal is to grow. As a result, we grow steadily bigger, stronger, more coordinated, more sexual . . . everything, no matter what. This default-to-grow signal sets up a tide of youth in our bodies, and almost everything gets better, willy-nilly. The tide of youth, man; it's sweet.

Then one morning, we wake up and notice that that tide has gone slack, and the morning after that it's on our nose. *Oh Lord!* The default signal has flipped over to decay. While biological aging actually starts in our thirties, most of us don't notice it until our forties or fifties. Now, every year we get steadily a little slower, weaker, less coordinated, more apt to get sick or fall down, less sexual, and grumpier. It is the worst. A tide of aging sets in, and it is relentless. It is working 24/7 to sweep you up on the rocks, where the crabs and the gulls are waiting to eat your big fat gut . . . Yucko!

But here's another great discovery of recent times: The tide is *not* that strong. If we are clever—and we are—we can consciously send some "grow signals" over that same signaling system. As Harry has already told you, you can *overcome 70 percent of normal American aging, until almost the end of life.* You can be roughly the same woman or man you were at forty-five or fifty until you are eighty and beyond. Best news in centuries! Some stuff is on the biological time line and you can't do a lot about it; your libido goes to hell (sob!), and your maximum heart rate goes down regardless. You get a little weaker and slower. That's why there are almost no professional athletes over forty—too bad. But *c'mon*! Seventy percent of aging is in our own hands! You can't play shortstop for the Yankees anymore. But you're *mostly yourself* still, and you will be for another forty years or so. That's huge!

Here is something better: The same physical messages we send by being active can eliminate an astonishing 50 percent of all serious illnesses and accidents after, say, age forty. Think about that:

THE DOCTOR IS IN: Decay Is Optional

There's a critical distinction between aging and decay. There is *a* biology of aging that you can't do anything about: Your hair gets gray, your heart rate declines, your skin goes slack. But most of what we call aging and dread about getting older is actually decay. We are stuck with real aging, but decay is optional. You do not have to act or feel old.

A lot of people unconsciously assume that they will get-old-and-die: one phrase, almost one word, and certainly one seamless concept. That when they get old and infirm, they will die soon after, so a deteriorating quality of life does not matter. *That is a deeply mistaken idea and a dangerous premise for planning your life.* In fact, you will probably *get-old-and-live.* You can get decrepit, if you like, but you are likely to live for a long, long time, whether you like it or not. Many of you will live well into your nineties, whether you are in great shape or shuffling along on walkers. *How* you live those years is largely under your control.

There is not a medicine or a medical protocol that comes vaguely near it. We are talking about *eliminating . . . not putting off, but eliminating . . .* half of all the serious illnesses and accidents that the other kids are going to have, including heart attacks, strokes, many cancers, diabetes, and—the one I always forget—Alzheimer's. And falls, too. You don't realize how horrible falls are until you get a little older but, believe me, falls kill. And Harry says that both those numbers are conservative—too low, if anything.

What's the Secret Signal?

So what's the signal that's going to work this miracle? I wish I could say that it is mostly a matter of sitting in a darkened room, watching football on TV, and drinking bourbon out of a jelly jar. Or playing video games. But that is not the way it turns out.

The master signal for health, optimism, energy, effectiveness, and *youth . . .* is serious exercise, six days a week, until the day you die.

Huh! Pity. A design flaw, some would say. When Harry first told me that, I was a little taken aback and asked, "What's the deal?" The short answer is that no one really knows. But Harry speculates, with considerable confidence, that it is because we were designed, in the Darwinian crucible of survival, to function as *endurance predators.* We were designed to trot along beside the herds of buffalo and elands and such for hours at a time. We weren't as fast as the animals, but we had great focus and great endurance. When a buffalo faltered, why, we'd smack him on the head and eat him. Funny way to make a living, you may say today, but that is what we are built for. And we are astonishingly powerful and well-adapted machines for that purpose. Neither your physical brain nor your body has changed in millennia, and they think we are still out there, on the plains, chasing the dear old eland. Indeed, as long as we continue to function as endurance predators and *move*, the machine works wonderfully well.

Trouble is, we've mostly gone out of the endurance-predator racket and we're now *bone idle*, which is nice in a way. There were an awful lot of thorns and other crap out there on the savanna. And rotten weather and rival predators (*lions*, for God's sake). Conversation was not amusing. So it is good to come inside and fool with computers and flirt with coworkers instead. And we can hope that, in a few million years, our bodies will adapt to the new dispensation, and that's all we'll have to do. But not in your lifetime, sweetheart, and certainly not in mine. And in idleness, our bodies get hugely confused. And fall apart. Atrophy, sickness, depression . . . on and on and getting worse every stinking year. Dreadful.

How Much Exercise Did You Say?

The answer is, six days a week, forty-five to sixty minutes a day. Sounds horrendous, but it is actually a terrific deal because the decay signals are running, nonstop, 24/7, and they are very effective. After age forty you lose up to 10 percent of your muscle mass a decade, and the same is true for bone mass, as well as for coordination and balance. The amazing news is that we are able to reverse all that—over 70 percent of it anyway—by moving, doing physical exercise a measly forty-five to sixty minutes a day, six days a week. How come we get away with so little exercise? Well, there is a cascade of grow signals while you actually work out. Then there is an "aura" period that lasts for hours afterward when the grow signals continue. And that's all you need. Interestingly, you get as much health and fitness benefit from one hour as you are going to get. More is not better. Harry and I think it makes sense to have one long day a week when you go hiking or biking for a couple of hours at a modest pace, but in general the daily forty-five to sixty minutes will do just fine. And doing that is much, much easier and more fun than you might think.

What Do You Actually Do?

There are two basic categories of exercise, and it is critical that you do both of them in the course of a week, because they do very different things for you. It is also key that you do the warm-ups for about ten minutes before you work out. (I hate to warm up, but I do these religiously because they help preserve range of motion and flexibility and fight off stiffness that can come with aging.) The most important exercise is *aerobic activity*; that's biking or swimming or doing the treadmill or the rowing machine to get your heart rate up and keep it there for about forty-five minutes. We'll get into the details in a minute.

Almost as urgent, but *for entirely different reasons*, is *strength training*, which you should do two days a week. Strength training has the most impact on your *quality of life*, and it is where almost all of us need to learn the most (and unlearn dumb stuff). It is also the hardest to learn to do right, and why this book will be particularly helpful. Because Bill Fabrocini is so good.

All exercise is hugely important, but none is more important than aerobic exercise. Which is where we go next.

CHAPTER TWO

The Magic Bullet: Aerobic Exercise

f there were a magic bullet in this life—and there is not—but if there were, it would be aerobic exercise. It is the flywheel of the good life. Because it does five amazing things that nothing else can do. And the five include some of the most important things in your life. Strength training is hugely important, too, but we can do only one thing at a time.

Five Amazing Things Aerobics Do for You

1. Aerobic exercise rebuilds and strengthens your aerobic base, the system that brings fuel and oxygen to the teeny engines (the mitochondria) in your muscles where they are "burned" so you can move. The same system takes away the waste products—lactic acid and so on—after the "burn," which is just as important. (The pain when you run out of steam and feel as if you are out of breath actually comes from the buildup of lactic acid, not muscle pain or lack of air. Huh!) And you, Beloved Reader, almost certainly need rebuilding pretty badly, because the likelihood is that you don't begin to get enough exercise. And in all that idleness, your aerobic base has gone to hell. Do you notice it? Of course you do. You get out of breath going up one flight of stairs. You shrink from the idea of walking five blocks. You don't feel like yourself. Stuff like that. It seems minor and temporary but it is not. You know why?

Because it is rot and it is never going away unless you do something major about it. Indeed, it is going to get steadily worse and worse until you are flat-out crippled by it. Being able to *move* is who you are, in nature. If you cannot move freely, you will be eased out of the herd, even if your herd is respectable-looking men and women from work and your neighborhood. Being able to move runs deep. Not being able to move takes you out of the game and makes you a dope. Sorry.

What went wrong? That's easy: In idleness, the little engines, the mitochondria, die off by the million. Your "horsepower" drops sharply. Very sharply. The capillaries that carry food and oxygen to the little engines (and carry away the ashes afterward) dry up and close, and . . . your horsepower drops some more. And the same rot has extremely creepy side effects. But here's the short version: In idleness, the whole system goes to hell, with disastrous consequences.

The great news is that aerobic exercise cures rot. Aerobic exercise *restores and repairs* the aerobic system; it gets you moving again. Pretty darned fast, too. You get millions of new mitochondria, vast new networks of capillaries. In a surprisingly short time, you feel better and are much more able to move freely. You start to feel like a human being again and not like a busted-down old plop. You start to feel like yourself.

2. Aerobic exercise reduces disease. Aerobic exercise radically reduces inflammation, which means it eliminates 50 percent of the worst diseases in our lives forever. It's much more complicated than this, but inflammation is the Great Satan inside our bodies. That is a simplification, but it is true: Inflammation is your mortal enemy. So let me say it again because it won't sink in the first time: By reducing inflammation, serious aerobic exercise *eliminates* 50 percent of the worst diseases. Modern medicine is amazing, but there is nothing in all of medicine that comes close to that.

Here, much simplified, is how it works. In the normal course— when you are sitting at your desk or watching TV and your blood is barely trickling around your body—your blood itself is mildly inflammatory. Your own precious blood is making things a little bit worse, with its slow, steady drip of inflammation. But when you do serious aerobic exercise, you *change the chemistry of your blood*, and it becomes anti-inflammatory. It becomes a powerful, healing balm, coursing through your body, making things radically better.

3. Aerobic exercise improves your mood and reduces depression. Depression is a bear in this country; it ruins lives, makes you a loser at work, ends careers, all kinds of dreadful stuff. It's gotten better with antidepressant drugs, but they are not perfect. It's hard to get the dosage right. There are side effects. *You* change and you have to change the dosage to fit, which is not always easy. But good news: Recent scientific studies support the observed fact that serious aerobic exercise is the single best thing you can do to combat depression and raise mood.

It is the best kind of "mood medicine." And we are not just talking about the "runner's high." We are talking about raising the water table of your mood in general. And that is good news for everyone, not just those with depression issues. It makes all of us more energetic, more optimistic, more decisive, and more effective. It is the secret sauce that makes us *younger next year*. In fact—big secret—if you jump on it right now, it can make you significantly younger *this year*. Could happen.

4. Aerobic exercise reduces stress. I think of stress as "the Corporate Sickness" in this country. Stress, unease, anxiety is the constant companion of so many of us at all levels of society. And it's not just unpleasant, it is debilitating: It saps our energy and effectiveness, a lot like depression. It makes us less effective while it is making us wretched. Even more seriously, it is making us *sick*. Chronic stress releases inflammation into the bloodstream . . . the Great Satan inside our bodies.

Businesspeople tell me all the time that they do not have enough time to work out. *Puh-lease!* People who exercise steadily have less stress; they use their time much more effectively. They have *more time*, not less. Try it and see if it makes a difference in a couple of weeks.

5. Aerobic exercise makes you smarter. As Harry wrote in the Introduction, scientific research in the last decade has shown that aerobic exercise grows new brain. You get 10 percent more cognitively efficient. Our old belief was that we were given a certain number of marbles ("brain cells" as we thought of them then) at birth, and we started to lose them at about age thirty-two. And when they were gone, there were no more. False. We get new brain cells all the time. They pop up, have a look around, and see what's going on. If you are watching daytime TV, they shrug and die a quick death. But if you are leading an active, engaged life and using your mind, why the new brain cells jump right in and go to work, just like the old ones. And sure enough, the only way to increase their output—aerobic exercise. Oh.

Where Do I Start?

Let us assume, just for fun, that you are not a complete buffoon and that we have piqued your curiosity. Indeed, you are thinking about jumping on it, big time, sometime soon. Excellent. Now the natural question arises, what do I have to do? And where do I start? Up to you, of course, but here's one idea. Sit down with a pad and pen and make some notes. You're going to be at this for a while, so it makes sense to plan a little. Maybe write down some vague goals for a year from now, or five years: how you'd like to feel, what you'd like to be able to do that you can't do now . . . maybe what you want to weigh. How you want to be at work

---

♺ DOCTOR'S ORDERS: Don't Skip This Box

This is not pro forma advice; it is from Dr. Henry S. Lodge himself. See *your* doctor before you embark on any of this. It is possible, at your age, that you have a condition you're totally unaware of that could make a sudden, new exercise program a grave threat. Don't take the chance. By now, you should be seeing your doctor once a year anyway. Bottom line: No matter how fit you are, check with your doctor and ask if you need a stress test before you start a serious exercise regimen.

. . . what kind of guy or girl. Your "image" and all that. Don't go nuts—it's just a device to motivate you and make this more fun. Just daydream for a bit about how good things might be.

Next make a list of aerobic activities that you like. Or at least can stand. In the next chapter we'll go into more detail about the different kinds. It is important to find one or two you like; it makes it so much easier. And don't hesitate to include stuff you don't do now like cross-country skiing or even rowing. Who knows? Then, if you feel like it, make yourself a little note about how important this is—or is not—to you. Don't be shy: No one is going to see it.

And here is some radical advice: Whatever great or rotten shape you're in right now, commit for the next month, anyway, to do some kind of aerobic exercise six days a week. Soon we'll switch over to strength training on two of those days. But it is the six-day structure that matters now. If you're in awful shape, do much less on a given day. But change your clothes and do something—even if it's for fifteen minutes only—six days a week. Get that structure in your head.

MAKE IT YOUR JOB. One of the best pieces of advice you are ever going to get goes like this: Think of exercise as your new job. Go to your gym the way you go to work. You don't decide every day whether or not to go to work, you just go. It's one of the most important things you learned in the workplace: *Use it now.* If you are older and partly retired, this is even more important. You need the structure. And, frankly, you need it even more than younger people because the *tide of aging* gets stronger as we get older; we need the *grow* signals even more. So make it your job.

One useful trick for some people is to have a schedule. Write your exercise "appointment" in your calendar and don't let anything or anyone intrude on it. Schedule a regular time—first thing in the morning is best for me—when you change into your duds and head off to the gym or pool. No one has the character to make a fresh decision every day to go to the gym. Go on "automatic" or you'll quit. Harry has worked on this with thousands of patients, and it's the habit and routine of exercise that lead to success.

Start Slow

S tart slow. Slower than what feels good. And hold at that level until you get your feet under you. Start out by pushing yourself hard enough to sweat, but at a level that matches your current fitness. Remember, we're talking about being younger next year, not younger tomorrow. Feel your way. You are a slightly old guy/girl now. You have Blacky Carbon and Gummy Sludge in your circulatory system. And your muscles and joints are not ready to go full bore.

FIRST DAY: After the warm-up, slowly increase the pace of your biking or using the treadmill or whatever you're doing, and get your heart rate up to 60 to 65 percent of your max and level off. (See page 29 to figure out your maximum heart rate.) Keep it up for ten or fifteen or twenty minutes that first day, whatever is comfortable. Cool down for a few minutes. Maybe do some stretches. Go home. You have just started the sacred process of building your aerobic base, adding a few mitochondria, stringing a few new capillaries, sending some new signals to your whole body. Nice work. Very nice work.

SECOND DAY: Do the same thing. If the first day knocked you sideways, do less. If you feel pretty good, do more. Keep inching along at the long-and-slow level with your heart rate at 60 to 65 percent of your maximum, (see "How to Calculate Your Maximum Heart Rate" on opposite page) for all of the first week and maybe for much longer. Your goal is to do forty-five minutes of Long and Slow aerobic exercise without any discomfort. You should be able to keep your heart rate at 60 to 65 percent, say, during a bike ride or hike while carrying on a conversation. If, at the end of the first week or the second or the third, you still cannot go this hard for forty-five minutes, that's fine. Just keep on keeping on. There's no rush. Building your aerobic base is the most important aspect of this regimen. It's okay if it takes a while.

Final bit of boring advice: Write stuff down. This helps some people more than others, but it helps everyone some. Write down every day what you did. Keep track of your progress. Shorthand is fine. Give yourself the idea that *someone* is keeping track, *someone* cares. Even if it's only you.

Last word: This won't be possible for a lot of you but, if you have a spouse or good pal who cares about this stuff, get him or her involved. It is so much easier to exercise with someone else. My wife, Hilary, and I do virtually all of this together. Think that helps? Oh yes.

I hope that exercise is fun for you. Or that it becomes fun for you, as it has for me. And for God's sake don't feel guilty because it is *too much fun*. I am blessed with the kind of disposition that sees the good side of things and enjoys stuff. Hooray for me. But increasingly I have come to believe that being happy and having fun is subject to "manipulation," too. You can make up your mind to be upbeat. And damned if it doesn't happen. Every time? Of course not. But it works surprisingly well. Give it a shot.

There you go. Do some aerobic exercise four days a week for two weeks. Then two months. Then the rest of your life. Congratulations!

How to Calculate Your Maximum Heart Rate

If you are going to be doing aerobic exercise for the rest of your life, it might not be a bad idea to have some sense of how *hard* you are working out. Your heart rate is *the best measure* of aerobic intensity; it tells you everything. And the best way to know your heart rate is to get and use a heart rate monitor.

Go to a sports store and buy the simplest one they have. A heart rate monitor is a two-part gizmo—a strap that goes around your chest and a wristwatch that goes around your (duh) wrist. The strap picks up the electric signal sent out every time your heart beats and transmits it to the little watch. Once it starts to pick up the beat (it often takes a while), look down and there is your heart rate.

Pretty soon, you are going to want to know what percent of your "maximum heart rate" that number on the little watch represents. *That* is what this is all about. To figure out your own max, use this simple formula: Take 70 percent of your age and subtract that number from 208. The result is the best *estimate* of your maximum heart rate. Thus, I am eighty (not my fault: I have a note from Harry); 70 percent of that is 56. I subtract that from 208 and come up with an estimated max of 152. If you are fifty, your estimated max will be 173.

Then figure out 60 percent, 65 percent, 70 percent, 80 percent, and 85 percent of your max with a pencil and paper. Memorize 'em or write 'em down. They'll come in handy. A day when you get to 60 percent of your maximum heart rate and stay there for about thirty minutes is a day you are working out.

Because individuals vary a lot, no formula is accurate for everyone. My real max is 165, not 152, for example. The only *real* answer is to find your *real* max. Wait until you are in really good shape, then do some serious exercise, like intervals, until your heart rate is up near 90 percent of your max. Stop before you think you have to and look at your heart rate monitor. *The highest number you see* is your actual max. (Actually, since you stopped a bit short of the hardest you could go, add five points and call that your actual max.)

CHAPTER THREE

"It's Been Awhile . . ."

Suppose that you are part of the 99 percent of the population that has not been working out pretty hard, six days a week, for the last few years. Indeed, let us postulate that, if you tried to ride a bike or do the elliptical at a sweat-inducing, hard-breathing clip for forty-five minutes or an hour, (a) you probably couldn't do it and (b) if you could, you'd be a mess for a week. We understand that. People do go to hell, in idleness. Most of us *have already gone to hell in idleness*, so don't feel uneasy and don't feel like a jerk. You are not a jerk. The whole country is ridiculous, but that's another matter. *You* are a shining star in this sea of dopes because *you* have decided to do something about it. And as scary as it may look at the outset, it is not all that hard.

But it sure does look it, and sometimes feel it. I am quite a fit old chap these days, but I was not when Harry and I first dreamed up this ridiculous six-day rule. Uh-uh. I was not a mess, like many of Harry's new patients, but not amazing either, believe me.

John on the Beach

One of my favorite stories about starting out on an exercise program involves a patient of Harry's, a guy we'll call "John on the Beach." John was in his sixties, about to retire to Florida, and an appalling mess. He was a hundred pounds overweight, he was in hideous physical shape, he hated his wife, hated his job, hated everything. He dreaded the idea of going to Florida.

Harry saw him just before he left New York and was blunt: Get a serious exercise habit, Harry said, or you will die. John on the Beach heard that (which was a blessing; not everyone can hear that dire warning) and, as soon as he got to his place near the beach in Florida, he went for a half mile walk in the soft sand. Hey . . . good for him. But the next day he felt as if he had been hit by a truck. He could barely get out of bed. That was too hard a start for a guy like John. But God bless him, he struggled to his feet the next morning, took some aspirin, and went back out on the beach: walked a hundred yards. The next day, the same thing: a hundred yards. Then six days a week for the rest of the year, with more distance all the time. At the end of the year, he was walking five miles a day in the soft sand, he had lost sixty pounds, his vital signs were radically improved, and he looked and felt like a different man. And he was *happy*. Here, of course, is the moral: It doesn't matter where you start; it matters that you keep it up. Forever. Because *then* it will work. Like gangbusters.

THE DOCTOR IS IN: Long and Slow Aerobic Exercise

Light aerobic exercise is Long and Slow exercise at an easy pace—up to 70 percent of your peak heart rate. At this level, your muscles burn mostly fat, so it's your most fuel-efficient pace, the one you can keep up for a long haul—for those times when speed doesn't count, but mileage does. You might think it's a waste of time to exercise in this zone, but it's a wonderful pace. This is the metabolic zone where your body and brain heal and grow. Long, slow exercise is the opposite of the chronic inflammation of modern living. It's the tide of youth.

Let's take a morning walk on the beach to see how it goes. Sand between your toes, early morning sun coming off the water. Give yourself five minutes of slow, relaxed strolling to warm up, and then ease into a good, stiff walk for about twenty minutes. You're taking it easy, and your muscles are burning fat over a low flame. As you loosen up and start to hit your stride, the fat burns hotter and faster. When you hit about 70 percent of your heart's maximum output, your leg muscles are working at the upper limit of their low aerobic zone. ("Aerobic" means your muscles have all the oxygen they need.) You can go all day, but you can't go fast.

Well, it turns out you don't have to for the health and longevity benefits we're talking about, because you've walked steadily into C-10 (or repair) territory. This all happens automatically through a carefully choreographed chemical dance within your bloodstream and body. Long, slow exercise builds your muscles, heart, and circulation; mobilizes your fat stores; and then goes beyond that to let your body heal. You become more fit with harder exercise, but you gain more endurance and general healthiness with prolonged light exercise.

Harry and I could tell you a hundred stories like that . . . a thousand. The amazing thing about the book *Younger Next Year* is that it truly has changed lives. This book may change yours. Go for it.

The simple point of this story is that you rebuild your aerobic base simply by using it. What that means is that you can run (or ski or hike or bike) harder and faster, and do it for much longer. You are an "aerobic predator" whether you want to be or not. It is what you were designed for. With exercise, you become a much, much better one. You become "more yourself."

For a long time, people thought that we—like car engines— literally wore out with use. We had only so many revolutions or whatever before we wore away the "piston walls" and died. But no! We are living flesh, and it doesn't work that way. When we use our bodies, we do not wear the system down, we build it up. Indeed, that is the only way to make it stronger. With aerobic exercise, you increase the horsepower of the whole machine. Use it and it grows. Let it sit idle and it rots.

How much can you rebuild? Plenty. I have been a wretched athlete all my life, but I am skiing the double black diamonds in the winter. Far better skiers than I quit decades ago. I can comfortably bike eighty miles (Harry and I are going to do one hundred miles in the Berkshire Hills this spring). I can row pretty hard for three miles, and so on. You may not want to do any of that stuff, which is fine. But you can, if you like. Because you will have the critical aerobic base for it. Because *this stuff works*.

So What Kind of Exercise?

Okay, you're still asking, "So what do I do?" Well, you start with aerobics (and stay with all aerobics for all six days, the first week . . . perhaps the first month . . . gotta bring up your aerobic base to be able to do strength training). You pick one or two aerobic activities off what is a pretty long and attractive menu. And it doesn't matter which one, as long as *you* like it, or can at least stand it. And you may want to bear in mind that aerobic exercise is seriously addictive. It becomes more attractive as you do it, and—after a while—you feel bad when you go without. That's a break.

Join a Gym

If you can bear it—and some people cannot—it makes a ton of sense to join a gym. It doesn't have to be fancy—the Y is fine. This is a big step and an important one. We have said that exercise is "your new job," which is absolutely right. Well, the gym may be the new office for a lot of you. It helps to have someplace to go. It gives your exercise life structure. We will talk about the supreme importance of exercising outdoors, whenever possible, but there are plenty of times when that doesn't work. Then you want a gym. Also, gyms have trainers, which may be critical for you (we'll come back to that), and classes of various kinds.

Aerobic machines (and TV sets to watch while using them) are one of the big attractions of joining a gym. A lot of people like the endurance machines at the gym: the treadmills, stationary bikes, stair-climbers, skiing machines, and the like. This makes sense: They're easy to use, it's easy to regulate the "dosage," and the process is bearable for most. The simple treadmill seems to be the most popular, but here's a hint: I think you do best to crank up the angle of the treadmill a ways and get your exercise by "walking up a steep hill," rather than trying to trot or run on the flat. Better workout for your leg muscles, less jarring on your joints, especially your knees, and you get a serious cardio workout much sooner.

My favorite is the elliptical machine with arms for an upper body workout, and my next favorite is the rowing machine. There is a world of these gadgets out there, they get better all the time, and one of them is almost certainly going to suit you.

Classes count, too, and gyms have lots of them. Think spin classes; Zumba and other dance or step classes; yoga (which is generally closer to strength training but can be aerobic, too); "pump" classes, which combine strength training and aerobics; ski preparation classes . . . all kinds of stuff. Classes are great, if you're the type, because they feel good. And you always do more in groups than you do alone. I go to a lot of spin classes; one reason is that—for intervals—I always work harder in spin class than alone on the road. Pathetic but true.

My wife, Hilary, loves yoga, as do a lot of her pals (more women than men). All aerobic exercises are more or less created equal. Find your passion.

THE DOCTOR IS IN: On Yoga

Once you're fit and pretty strong, you might try yoga. Whereas weights build specific muscle groups in isolation, yoga integrates strength and balance training. The rich sensory stimulation of using muscle groups in different combinations, and linking this with breathing, mind exercises, and stretching, creates a more profound neurosensory and proprioceptive integration than Western exercise. You have to be reasonably fit to start yoga; after all, it was created by people who were already living a very physical life. Moreover, we have an aerobics class mentality that asks us to do more and better each day. If you do try yoga, think about starting with individual instruction for five sessions. The expense is well worth it, and if the instructor doesn't teach you how to listen to your body, find someone else. Group yoga classes, once you understand the basics, are among the best deals around, going for ten bucks in most places.

The Joy of Yoga

Twenty years ago I fell down a flight of stairs and broke my neck. The prognosis was pretty bad: I would steadily lose flexibility, range of motion, and strength; in short, I would become a near-cripple. None of that has happened, and I attribute some of my almost miraculous recovery to yoga—I did (and continue to do) yoga almost daily for rehab and maintenance. It was just what I needed to heal. This ancient practice explores and holds specific poses to build strength or it links poses in a choreographed flow that is a great aerobic workout. Yet no matter how rigorous or challenging the practice can be, yoga's ultimate goal is to become still—to focus on the breath and on the present moment. This meditative quality is sadly missing from most of our lives which, I suspect, is another reason that yoga is so appealing.

Yoga is often hard, never perfect, and always a joy as you realize that these poses have been designed and refined over centuries to refresh and strengthen your body and your mind. It takes a long time to develop the simple strength or flexibility to do some poses. If you are older—or if, like me, you have had a serious injury—you may never get to some of the more complicated ones. Never mind: It will do wonders at the level that is right for you. —HILARY COOPER

You hate gyms? You think you're going to look like an idiot in those Lycra costumes or whatever? You think that all those young hard bodies are going to sneer at you? Don't worry about it. For three reasons. First, you are not here to get dates; you're here to save your life, so the hell with them. Second, people are remarkably tolerant of older people who work out. They can only *hope* that they are working out when they are your age. Finally, people in gyms are apt to be a bit focused on their own workouts. They will not see you. They have their job, you have yours: Do it.

So take a deep breath, hold your nose if you have to, and join a gym. Eventually—as far-fetched as this sounds now—you may come to see this as a place you love to "get away" to, the scene of some of your happiest hours. Weird, I know, but true.

Go Outdoors

Whenever you can, go outside and do stuff in nature. We're talking biking, hiking, running, or rowing. You can do versions of all those things in the gym, but it is *so* much better to do them outside.

First, the technical reasons. When you ride a real bike on real roads, or hike up a trail, to say nothing of going for a row or cross-country skiing, you have to do a lot of balancing, just to stay upright. You have to use hundreds of tiny muscles and make thousands of mini-adjustments to avoid the rocks in the road, to keep the single scull even. In the gym, the machines do all that for you. And those critical small muscles tend to atrophy. So, exercising outside is almost always better for you.

Try a Healing Sport

Some sports, like tennis, pull you apart because they're centrifugal. Others, like running, beat on your joints remorselessly. For the lucky few who can still jog or run without pain, it's a delight. Go for it. But default to the low impact sports in the long run.

But a few sports actually knit you together. Your muscles and especially your joints feel better when you're done than when you began. Because they are low impact, most of us can do these forever. Biking is peculiarly like that. Swimming, cross-country skiing, the elliptical machine, and rowing, too. They are the "healing sports," and you ought to have at least one of them in your repertoire.

A Word About Bikes and Safety

If you haven't biked for a while, you may want to remind yourself that you are forty or fifty or sixty, not twenty, and that you have to be a hair more cautious. Wear a helmet all the time. I still bike in New York City traffic, but frankly, it's starting to scare me. If you're just getting back into the sport, I'd start someplace pretty calm and bucolic. And as with skiing or any "movement" sport, look around a lot more than you used to. Be predictable. Go in predictable lanes, and don't veer off without making damn sure there is no one behind you. Interesting point: Most people worry about overtaking cars. In fact, they cause very few biking accidents: It is usually other bikes or turning cars. Not as scary, but more deadly.

BIKING, THE IDEAL AEROBIC SPORT: It's great for you, it's low impact and safe for your knees, and you can do it until you are very old. Here are three more selling points about my favorite sport: (1) You already know how to do it. (2) It's wildly good for you. (3) It's great for your legs. Later on, we make the point that building up your legs is particularly important in the Third Act. Failing legs are what can put you on the walker or in the chair. When in doubt, default to exercise that helps your legs. Like bicycling.

When I ride a real bike outside, my heart rate routinely goes 15 percent higher than it usually goes in spinning class. Not because I'm trying harder, but because real biking is a little harder—and thus a little better for you. There's more going on. There's all that balancing all the time, all that looking around at the real world to see where you are and what's coming up. And there are those millions of tiny adjustments every minute to take account of the real world and balance and Lord knows what else. That stuff takes energy. And it's super for you. It brings all those pesky neurotransmitters back to life and makes them strong.

There is no machine more beautiful, more perfect in the form-follows-function line, more ideally suited to your purpose than the bicycle. You can get a good road bike, with modern gearing and brakes, for a few hundred bucks. If you're more or less a beginner, you may want to get a user-friendly "combination" bike—a bike with slightly fatter tires and that allows you to sit upright. They are less expensive, easier to ride, and a good way to reintroduce yourself to the sport. They still have great gearing and brakes, and they will give you more exercise, if anything. Oh, and get good biking shorts. And a comfortable seat.

Some people fear and dread biking and always will. "Riding around on a dangerous paper clip" one guy said to me, dismissively. Hey, if you feel that way, the hell with it. Some people just

---

⚕ THE DOCTOR IS IN: The Chemistry of Exercise

Remember, your body craves the *daily* chemistry of exercise. Whether the exercise is long, slow, and steady (an hour or two of good, hard walking) or shorter and more intense (running, swimming, or using the exercise machines at the gym) is a lot less important than the "dailyness" of it. So experiment with a variety of aerobic exercises at the gym and find some outdoor sports that you like: biking, kayaking, downhill or cross-country skiing, or stiff hiking. You might decide to keep your heart rate in the high aerobic zone (70 to 80 percent of your maximum heart rate) at the gym and in the low aerobic zone while exercising outside or vice versa. Whichever, you'll get great results. Remember that the whole point is to give your body and brain the sustained signals that tell them to grow younger. All forms of aerobic exercise produce C-6 in proportion to the duration and intensity. About one hour after exercising, C-10 will automatically flood your body.

don't like biking because they say it makes their butt hurt, and they will never be persuaded that that's temporary (it is). Others think it looks dangerous. Maybe, but I've never had a bad fall.

SWIMMING: The most important thing is to mix up the modes of exercise so you don't get bored. If you haven't gone swimming lately, give it a shot. Swimming is cheap and easy to do. And if you go at it with some energy, it's great aerobic exercise. Swim fans often say it's the perfect exercise, and we can see why. You use almost every muscle in your body, it's aerobically demanding, and it also stretches you out in a healthy way, like yoga. My daughter Ranie is crazy about swimming. Here's her version of the joy of this sport in open water:

The Joy of Swimming

You may have to be crazy to get to my level of the sport—to swim in the ice, or around Manhattan, the Straights of Gibraltar, or the English Channel, all things that I have done in my fifties. But open-water swimming in general is fantastic for anyone. I got into it some ten years ago, at a wonderful club on San Francisco Bay. And it has been my major sport—and a source of remarkable camaraderie. Swimming is superb exercise. There is no "pounding or twisting," and you can do it forever. It is often a group activity, which makes it more fun and more sustainable. Clearly, I have drunk my father's Kool-Aid. Maybe a drop too much. But do try swimming—especially open-water swimming. It is a great form of aerobics. —RANIE CROWLEY

CROSS-COUNTRY SKIING: If you're anywhere near snow, do not miss cross-country skiing. Even if you've never done it before. For one thing, it's bone-easy. After exactly one day, you'll be doing

The Joy of Cross-Country

It snowed like crazy up here in the Berkshires recently. I took one look out the window to check the temperature, then bustled down to the cellar and put on my cross-country ski gear. The snow is deep and light and I have to "break trail" along the old logging road that leads to the first of the huge, open fields that are the object of this journey. These fields—half a dozen of them—run for miles, north to south, and you rarely see a house, or even a barn. They are great, rolling farmlands, broken up by lines of windbreak trees every few hundred yards. Each is beautiful in a different way. But the most striking thing is the view of the Berkshires, a few miles away. These are not like my beloved Rockies, but the proportions are perfect and they are stunning.

The movement of cross-country skiing—the hard push-off on one foot, with one pole, and then the easy glide—is one of the nicest in sport. Very much like rowing—the hard catch and pull, then the slow and silent glide as the oars slide back. You can't really describe this stuff; you have to experience it. But that rhythm of push and glide, in near perfect silence, . . . well, it's worth anything. This is the Long and Slow pace, by the way (we'll talk in the next chapter about different paces, but this is the easy one); I am not working terribly hard. My heart rate mostly does not go above seventy beats a minute. You learned earlier from Harry that this is as hard as you ever have to work to get almost all the *health benefits* of an aerobic workout. It is a joyous pace, and you have plenty of time and energy to look around and soak up the beauty.

fine. It is a species of walking, after all. And once you get the hang of it, you can give yourself a massive dose of the very best aerobic exercise in some of the most beautiful places in the world. There is nothing better on earth than sliding gracefully along under trees heavily laden with fresh snow over the golf course in your hometown or up in the hills. The only sound the hiss of your own sweet skis and your breath. Sneak off alone and try it. You will thank me for the rest of your days.

Mix It Up

Find something you love, if you possibly can, and go for it. If you're lucky enough to have an athletic passion, by all means tap into it as a support for your exercise program. And try new stuff: You may surprise yourself. Don't miss a single chance to make

---

Kedging

Let's admit it. It's not easy to keep doing exercise six days a week, year in and year out. Sometimes we falter, sometimes we slip off the bike, we get bored, and sometimes we need help. We all do. So Harry and I have come up with just the thing: "kedging." Originally, it was a nautical term: When sailors were becalmed and drifting toward the rocks, they would literally pull themselves forward (using a small boat to set a small anchor) to get out of danger. They called kedging. It's what you have to do when you're tempted to say "the hell with it" and never exercise again. For our purposes, kedging means climbing out of the ordinary by setting a terrific goal for yourself (with a reward at the end) and working like crazy to get there. Make a long-range plan, maybe with a group of friends in some wonderful place, and then do it. It's demanding but fun, like signing up for a serious "adventure trip." Maybe one of those great bike trips in Europe, or a white-water rafting adventure, or a yoga retreat, or maybe a week at an interesting spa. Think about walking or running for a cause and get a friend to train with you. Most of these "kedges" mean training beforehand. But the training and anticipation perk us up and give shape and purpose to our daily training. And there's that great reward at the end.

this something you enjoy. Over time, you're far more likely to do stuff that's fun for you. I'm an expert on fun, I'd know.

And mix up your activities—to fight boredom and to use different muscle groups. This applies to everyone, no matter how fit you are. If you do nothing but bicycle, four days a week, for years, some of your muscles will be strong and your aerobics will be great. But some of your muscles that go unused will atrophy. As you get older, your body will get less and less tolerant of that kind of concentration. And you will wind up on the side of the road, in the gutter. That's what cross-training and whole-body movement is all about.

The Rich Hours

I f you're lucky, as I have been, then pretty soon aerobic exercise becomes one of the sweet places in your day. A time apart when you work hard but feel terrific (the wonderful "aerobic high") and draw a near-Zen-like satisfaction from your place in the world and in *movement*. That's a little fancy, but it's absolutely true, and it's something that is known to aesthetic souls and rough athletes alike. If you get into it, I predict that you will come to look forward to this time as a deeply personal treat. It's when I do some of my most creative thinking. And sometimes I just dope off. Nice. I am peculiarly in touch with myself at these times. It is an armature for meditation. I love it.

CHAPTER FOUR

How Hard
Should You
Work Out?

O ne of the questions that Harry and I get all the time is, "How hard do I work out when I'm doing aerobics?" The answer is, it depends. It depends, basically, on whether you are going to be satisfied with health on the one hand or eager to go beyond health to fitness on the other. There is a tendency to glorify fitness. Here is a tip: *Don't.* Because, for the vast majority of us, health is going to be all we ever want or need. It is a noble and deeply worthwhile goal. And it's simple. All you have to do to achieve the health benefits we've talked about (overcoming 70 percent of normal aging and eliminating 50 percent of serious illnesses) is work out for forty-five minutes to an hour at 60 to

LEVELS OF AEROBIC EXERCISE

ZONE	% OF MAX HEART RATE
Zone One (Long and Slow)	**60–70%**

This is a very fast walk or a modest run, for most people. You are breathing deeply but not panting. You can carry on a normal conversation. You feel you could do this for hours, once you're in decent shape. Chase down that antelope. This is as hard as many of you ever have to go for health.

Zone Two (Endurance)	**70–80%**

You are breathing deeply. You can still talk, but you're taking some deep breaths. You could do this for a while but not forever; not at the upper reaches, anyway. If you are in great shape, you can do this for a couple of hours. Zones One and Two are variations of the same thing; Zone Two is a more intense level One. Go there when you get in better shape and feel like it.

Zone Three (Interval)	**80–90%**

This is serious business. You are breathing pretty hard now. Talking is possible at the lower reaches of this level, but not at the upper ones. At upper levels you are panting hard. You can do this at the upper reaches for only a few minutes. You get to the upper reaches of this level only when you're in great shape. And your doctor knows what you're up to. This is fitness country. Mostly you do this level only for "interval" sprints of one to eight minutes, with rests in between. Remember: You never have to do this unless you feel like it.

Zone Four (Fight or Flight)	**90–100%**

I don't recommend going this hard for most people over sixty. This is flat-out. The lion or the robber is closing in, and you are giving it everything you've got. You can do this for only a short time, say, sixty seconds. Watch it! You can hurt yourself.

70 percent of your maximum heart rate, four days a week. (See "How to Calculate Your Maximum Heart Rate," page 29.) It may be a struggle to get there if you've been idle for a while, but eventually it is going to be easy. And the payoff is enormous.

But in our experience, a certain number of folks will want to go a little further. That may sound nuts to you now, but later on you may want to explore the world of *fitness,* which is a different kind of fun.

The table on page 45 may help as you read about different levels of aerobic exercise.

Long and Slow for Health

Aerobics for health means doing some kind of aerobic exercise at the 60 to 70 percent level, four days a week, for the long haul. And let me be clear, it is a deadly serious business, . . . a major achievement, I say. But describing it is easy. First, you warm up for ten to fifteen minutes (either with Bill Fabrocini's Preparation for Movement, page 90, or by doing some easy biking, swimming, the elliptical machine, or whatever you're up to that day). Then you gradually increase the pace or difficulty until you get to the 60 percent level. You stay there—or drift up as far as the 70 percent level if you feel like it—for, say, thirty minutes. Then cool down for five minutes, or go easy until your heart rate is back to normal. You're done.

Please do not be misled by the fact that this is so easy to describe. It is *not* easy to do. I am sorry to repeat myself but it is *so* important to stress that, if you get to this level and maintain it, you have done a wonderful thing that will profoundly change your life. Remember John on the Beach and his remarkable achievements? He never got beyond the Long and Slow Level.

Intensity for Health and Fitness

There may come a time when working out four days a week at the Long and Slow Level is too easy or comfortable. Then you may want to go further. Some of you are just going to "feel like it," out of sheer exuberance. If and when that cheerful day rolls around, congratulations.

What are the benefits of fitness? Get *fit* and your aerobic strength will be much, much greater. You will not just be able to walk a few miles with ease, you'll be able to jog or run. You won't just be able to bike firmly for ten or fifteen miles on level or rolling ground, you'll be able to bike the steep hills, go twenty miles routinely and fifty on special occasions. You will look for hills instead of avoiding them. The fitness level is great for weight control, too. And for some of us, it is major fun.

Endurance Aerobics

Okay, what's the next step, if you want to give fitness a try? Harry's and my advice is to move up gradually. Which is to say, first move into the Endurance Level of aerobic exercise. That is Zone Two on the table on page 45, or 70 to 80 percent of your max. It means you are breathing hard and sweating quite a bit. You can still talk, but not with complete ease.

I should probably say, at this point, that the quickest route to fitness, according to serious trainers, is to do intervals (discussed below) at a ferocious clip. But Harry's and my experience is that intervals are just too damned hard for most of us after age forty or fifty, so we don't do them. The beauty of exercise at the Endurance Level is that it is doable once we get in decent shape. Intervals are a torture for almost everyone, including serious athletes; they are supposed to be. But Endurance Level exercise is fun.

To do aerobics at the Endurance Level, first do your usual warm-up and then gradually bike (or ride the elliptical or whatever) harder and faster until your heart rate gets up into the 70 to 80 percent range. At this point you may want to pay closer attention to your heart rate monitor because it is easy to overestimate how hard you are working out. (The beauty of the nasty old monitor is that it doesn't let you lie to yourself.) As to whether you work out at the 70 or at the 80 percent range on an Endurance day, suit yourself. The harder and longer you go, obviously, the more fitness you will achieve.

One basic rule for fitness training is the same, regardless of the level of intensity you reach: *Do alternate days of hard and easy workouts*. That is, do one day at the Long and Slow Level (that never changes) because you need that time for recovery. You stress your muscles (and everything else) on the hard days, but you actually build and get stronger on the recovery days. So, one day of Long and Slow and one day of intensity. Then repeat.

In time you should be able to do Endurance aerobics for an hour or two, if you feel like it. And the payoff is that you'll achieve significantly more fitness than you will at the Long and Slow level. For a lot of us, that is as deep into fitness as we want to go.

Intervals

Okay, serious endurance athletes and their coaches think that doing intervals is the cat's whiskers, and I am sure they are right. Too much fun for me, most of the time. But if you want real fitness and want it pretty fast, try intervals. Though, I caution you, it ain't easy.

Harry asks me to make the point that this is a limited treatment of the complex subject of intervals. He says it will be detailed enough only for, say, 95 percent of you. Aww, rats! Only 95 percent of you. For the handful who want to go deeper, there is a lot more from Riggs and me in the book *Thinner This Year*. Or you may want to read Chris Carmichael (biking) or Rob Sleamaker. The latter's *Serious Training for Endurance Athletes* may make teeth ache a little bit (just a touch of detail), but it's good. If you get hooked to the point where you want to learn more, then Riggs and I have done our job.

First, as ever, you do warm-ups or some easy running or whatever at 50 to 60 percent of your max. Next get out a watch with a visible second hand and your heart rate monitor and time your intervals (the go-for-it stretches) and your slow or recovery stretches. Does this sound a little complicated? Well, it is. It's much easier if you have a coach to do the timing (and to yell at you to go faster), but most of us are on our own. It can be done but it takes some getting used to. I hate it.

After you have warmed up, then hit it pretty hard—not really flat-out, but hard—for 60 or maybe 120 seconds. That is the "interval," the hard part. Check your heart rate. On this first one, you may not reach 80 percent of your max. But it builds as you do successive intervals. Now go easy (65 to 70 perecent) for a minute or two. (These times are a bit arbitrary, and there are thousands of variations.) In the early stages, you'll want the intervals to be short (60 to 120 seconds) and the rest segments to be as long or longer. Then repeat. And repeat again. As you get into it, you may do longer intervals with shorter rest periods. We give you some samples to try on pages 51 to 52.

On your first few days, you'll do well to last for a total of fifteen minutes. You may be pooped before that, if you really hit it during the Interval part. A half hour of Interval Level is not shabby, even for a pretty fit athlete. Forty-five minutes of them and you are amazing. Be sure to cool down after an all-out effort like this. Cooling down, remember, is a simple matter of biking or whatever slowly until your heart rate comes down to about 50 percent of your max.

Caveat: It is important to use your heart rate monitor (see page 29) when you're doing intervals, so you'll know how hard you are hitting it. You know: Did I get to 80 percent? Am I getting too far over 90 percent? Stuff like that. Sadly, heart rate monitors—which I believe in with all my heart and head and liver—have a teeny flaw that makes them imperfect in the world of intervals: They have a little lag of five to twenty seconds between the time you change your level of effort (and thus, your heart rate) and the time it registers on the little watch. If you are doing thirty-second intervals, that eats into their usefulness some. But I wouldn't worry. All you really need to know is how high you went during the push. And from time to time you'll want to know how long it took your heart to calm down again. The monitor will tell you all that. You just have to get used to its little ways.

Four Interval Days

On Interval Level days you are trying to get your heart rate into the Interval Zone (80 to 90 percent of your heart rate) for one to ten minutes at a time. It means moving in and out of that zone from thirty to forty-five minutes a day on schedules like the ones below. These four Interval days (good for two weeks) were created by *Thinner Next Year* aerobics expert Riggs Klika to get you started. They go up a little in difficulty. The magic of intervals, says Riggs, is crossing and recrossing your "aerobic threshold" (which is in the low 80 percent range). Riggs does not specify, in these examples, what activity to pursue, because it doesn't matter. You can do intervals on a bike, an elliptical, or a rowing machine, your choice.

Caveat: You want to be in good shape before you try these. And work into it gradually.

#1

Warm-Up	1 x 10 minutes
Workout	5 x 30 seconds (80 to 90 percent of max heart rate) with 3-minute rest between intervals (complete rest, or very slow pace)
Warm-Down	1 x 10 minutes
Total Time:	approximately 37 minutes

Note: *If you can't do five intervals, do as many as you can today and simply take longer rest periods between the intervals you do.*

#2

Warm-Up	1 x 10 minutes
Workout	1 x 3 minutes (80 to 90 percent of max heart rate) with 2-minute rest between intervals
	1 x 2 minutes (80 to 90 percent) with 2-minute rest
	1 x 1 minute with 2-minute rest
	Perform the above set 2 times
Warm-Down	1 x 10 minutes
Total Time:	approximately 55 minutes

Note: *If this seems challenging, try only one set.*

#3

Warm-Up	1 x 10 minutes
Workout	3 x 3 minutes (80 to 90 percent of max heart rate) with 5-minute rest between intervals
Warm-Down	1 x 10 minutes
Total Time:	approximately 45 minutes

Note: *The extra rest should allow you to reach Zone Three each time.*

#4

Warm-Up	1 x 10 minutes
Workout	Ladder (explained on page 53): 1-2-3-4-3-2-1 minutes with 2-minute recovery between each interval (try to reach 80 to 90 percent of your maximum heart rate each time)
Warm-Down	1 x 10 minutes
Total Time:	approximately 50 minutes

Spin Class

If you want to try serious intervals but find the foregoing too daunting, think about a good spin class. A spin class (group rides on stationary bikes) can be a very serious Interval day, if the instructor is any good. And I find these classes curiously seductive and—more important—doable. Good leaders are apt to be very motivational. The loud music helps. As does the fact that you are doing it in a group. And yet *you* regulate the level of intensity. How hard you are really working out—in response to the instructor's urgings—is your secret.

A Rowing Machine or Scull Interval Day

Here's a great tip: The best machine for aerobic activity is the rowing (or erg) machine, a dry-land version of a single scull. It is better than the elliptical, the stationary bike, or the treadmill because it uses your whole body, especially your core. And it's harder because it engages almost all your muscle groups. Don't be put off by the difficulty—that's what makes it so great.

Harry was hurt that I did not mention his beloved NordicTrack machine in this list. He points out, correctly, that cross-country skiing is *the* most effective aerobic exercise, and he assumes that the NordicTrack is thus the best machine. Could be. I owned one, but didn't use it. There was a time when it seemed almost everyone owned a NordicTrack. Then they started to migrate to the attic, and then out to the curb, with a FREE sign beside them. If they have one flaw—and I may be alone in this view—it is that they are so boring that you might fall asleep while using one. But if you dodge that bullet, they work like a charm. Me, I love cross-country skiing in real snow and dread the machine. Need I say that Harry is a slightly more virtuous human being than I? And that he is a stranger to boredom? *Noble Harry!*

Here is a great Interval day for either the erg or an actual single scull. I got it from the Harvard rowing coach, Dan Boyne, when I was training for that incredible rowing race, the Head of the Charles. It's called a "ladder." You climb up. And you climb down. Then you lean over and vomit into the Charles River. Just kidding.

After a warm-up, take one hard stroke. Then one easy one. Then two hard strokes. Two easy ones. Keep it up all the way to 17 hard, followed by 17 easy. (Why 17? I have no idea.) You just climbed up the ladder. Now you climb down. Drop to 16 hard and 16 easy. Then 15 and 15 and so on, down to one. It takes only about a half hour but, at the end, you are whipped. If you can build a "ladder" for other aerobic activities you like, try it.

How High to Take Your Heart Rate During Intervals

The answer for most of us is probably 85 percent. And not more than 90 percent, even if you're pretty keen. The reason Riggs gives is interesting: Crossing the "aerobic threshold" is what does the trick of promoting fitness. And for most fit people, the aerobic threshold is at about 80 to 83 percent of your max. Cross that range, and you are doing the magic thing in the world of intervals. Really fit (and really young) endurance athletes take it higher, but I wouldn't if I were you. Harry and I would urge that, if you are in your fifties or sixties or older, you not go above 90 percent. You will get all the fitness you need at the 80 to 85 percent level. And there are increased risks above that level for heart attacks and such.

HEART ATTACKS, DID YOU SAY? People worry a lot about killing themselves by doing exercise, because it does happen once in a great while. But what you want to bear in mind, in general, is that being *idle* is far more dangerous than exercising. As always, Harry gets it just right: If you want to be as safe as possible for *one day*, he says, go home, lock the door, and get in bed. But, he goes on, that is just about the worst thing you can do, over time. So follow a sane but serious exercise regimen, and never go over 90 percent of your max without a serious talk with your doctor.

Half-Baked Intervals

confess that, most of the time, I satisfy myself with intervals that serious trainers would probably sneer at. The attraction? They are intervals. They will create fitness. And they are doable.

My favorite is one invented by my wife, Hilary. We call it "The TV Solution." Go to the gym and turn on the TV. During the substance of the show—movie, football, or whatever—go in Long and Slow mode. Then, during the commercials, do an interval. Pump your heart out. When it's over, slow down again. The beauty of it: You don't need a stopwatch, you don't have to watch the stupid commercials, and it is manageable (because the commercials are much farther apart than the intervals in a real interval program).

Another favorite is biking in the hills. If you're lucky enough to live in a hilly area, just do the obvious: Take it fairly easy on the flats and hit it hard on the hills.

And that, ladies and gentlemen, is the world of interval training.

Sometimes I do 'em, when I have an event or kedge I am building to. But I must confess that my default hard day is very apt to be at the Endurance Level, or my own easier version of intervals, like hill biking. Now that you know the range of options and the issues, you decide what you want your life to be and how much time you want to invest.

Here's my parting thought. Health is a blessing—all the blessing that most of us want. Fitness is a much bigger blessing, but you have to be a little bit crazy to pursue it. I *know* that people look at me, biking or skiing away in all weather, and whisper to one another, "That poor fellow has lost his mind." Could be, but it feels pretty neat. You might just want to try it. But quit if it's not worth it. Fitness is a luxury. Health is mandatory.

CHAPTER FIVE

Skip This Chapter

People who really get into aerobic exercise—and I mean *really* get into it—are fascinated by the details of just how the "aerobic machine" works at different fitness levels and at different intensities of exercise. This chapter goes into that somewhat. You may want to skip it now and come back later, because it's hard (read "boring"). I confess that I am fascinated by it, as are some of my pals who have really gotten into the *Younger Next Year* life. Up to you. But for heaven's sake, don't get stuck here. It is far more important that you do the exercises that follow than grind to a halt in all this science.

What we're talking about here is "different metabolic pathways that you access, to different degrees, with different levels of exercise intensity." Does that make you hot? Great—read on.

One of the miracles of the human body (and one of the keys to our success as endurance predators) is that we can burn two very different fuels and use two very different metabolic pathways. Yes, children, we can burn carbs (which are metabolized or digested into sugar by the time they are ready to burn) on the one hand or fat on the other. Before we get into that, here is a home truth that will help you understand everything better. It is something basic that a lot of smart people seem not to know. Everything we eat is carbohydrate, fat, or protein. And basically we don't burn protein. The body's engines are limited to burning carbs or fat. Period. Anyone who tells you to quit eating either carbs or fat is an idiot; we have to burn both. And you do burn both almost all the time. (Dropping the "bad" or refined carbs or trans fats is another matter; that's a good idea.)

Okay, back to the great, dual-track mystery. Most of what we eat turns into glucose or glycogen, which are both just forms of sugar. That includes all vegetables and fruit, all grains (both virtuous and not), sugar, the works. The rest turns into (or remains as) fat and protein. And remember, protein doesn't count as far as fuel is concerned. Some sugar gets stored in the muscle cells for immediate use (glycogen). Some is stored in the blood, and quite a lot in the liver. Like the glucose stored in muscles, this is easy to access. The rest is turned into fat. The body burns sugar and fat simultaneously all the time, but, in general, fat is harder to access. There is an almost endless supply of fat but it enters the bloodstream to be used as fuel pretty slowly. So when the body runs out of sugar, it more or less stops. *If* you are working out pretty hard and burning a lot of fuel. It's more complicated than that but not a lot.

As I say, you burn both fat and sugar (in one form or another), all the time. What changes dramatically (and importantly) is *the mix* of the two, as well as the ability of the body to access fat both earlier in the exercise process and deeper into intensity. (Hint: People who are in better shape can access fat more easily and burn more of it even at higher levels of intensity. That is just one reason they are so much cuter.)

Trainers and others used to talk lovingly about a "fat-burning zone." And the wonder was that the slower zone—the Long and Slow workout—was said to be that magical, fat-burning place. Sad news: There is no fat-burning zone. And if there were one, it would be flat-out, crazy Interval Zones at 90 to 100 percent of your max, not the Long and Slow. What *is* true is that you burn a higher *percentage* of fat versus carbs in Long and Slow mode. *But* you burn a higher absolute number of fat calories in intense exercise. Isn't that the worst? The people who work hardest get the most benefit. Sigh.

At 50 percent of your max, the ratio of fat to sugar in your fuel is about 50-50. You burn equal amounts.

At 60 to 80 percent of your max, you go to 80 percent sugar and 20 percent fat.

At 85 to 95 percent of your max, the mix is 95 percent sugar and 5 percent fat.

But remember this: No matter what, the absolute number of calories of fat burned goes up the harder you work out, regardless of these percentages. So, there is no fat-burning zone.

Burning fat is highly desirable for a bunch of reasons. First, it's terrible looking. Especially the fat around your gut, which is also a huge source of inflammation and, you know, sickness and death. Big fat piggies look awful and die young. How about that? More important to athletes, who are not apt to be overweight, there is an almost limitless supply of it. And that is true even if your percentage of body fat is, say, 12 percent, which is very lean indeed. As a practical matter you'll never run out. At all stages of athletic activity (or any other activity) you have to burn both sugar and fat, and eventually you are going to run out of sugar. Your body can't just switch over to fat when it runs out of sugar. It should, maybe, but it just doesn't work that way. When you run out of sugar, your body stops. Dead. You don't have that problem with fat.

So far this has been easy. Now it gets hard. Very hard. Turns out we have two very different metabolic systems. The main one—the aerobic system—burns fat and sugar *with oxygen*. The more exotic one—the anaerobic system—burns sugar with no oxygen at all (think of that!). The anaerobic system is absolutely wonderful for some uses. It burns hotter than the hinges of hell, and it is the optimal system for using your fast-twitch muscles (the ones you use for Fight or Flight) as opposed to the slow-twitch muscles (which you use for endurance activities). But it is a very messy "fire" and creates a lot of detritus, including lactic acid, which builds up super fast—way faster than the trash-removal system can get rid of it. Pretty soon, your muscles just cease to contract because of the buildup of "ashes," mostly lactic acid. You stop in major pain. You have hit The Wall. I have been there, lately, and it is bad. Agonizing, in fact. No one runs or rows through The Wall. Lactic acid rules.

You can go flat-out at a 100 percent anaerobic pace for thirty to sixty seconds. Actually, even that's an exaggeration. You have an *effective* burst of about seven seconds. Then you slow down appreciably, even if you are still in full anaerobic mode. Pure anaerobic stints are strictly fight-or-flight stuff. After a very short spurt, the lactic acid starts to build up and the muscles no longer work effectively.

Are you kids still there? Good, because we are coming to the payoff. The critical *threshold* in the body is not the point at which you go to 100 percent anaerobic effort (which you almost never do). No, the critical threshold—and the one that serious athletes and trainers talk and think about all the time—is the "lactate" threshold. *That* is the point at which the mix of stuff you burn is such that the ash from the fire, the lactic acid in particular, builds up faster than the exhaust system (your blood and your breath) can clear it away. Once you have crossed the lactate threshold, you can keep on going only so long before the buildup of lactic acid becomes intolerable and you stop.

If you are just barely over the lactate threshold, you may be able to go on for an hour or more. A lot more for great athletes. But eventually you'll stop. If you are *way* over that line, as in a flat-out sprint, you can do it for, say, only thirty to sixty seconds.

Who Cares?

Excellent question, and the answer is high-end endurance athletes who want to move a little faster and go a little longer without hitting The Wall. The weird and wonderful thing is that athletes can *move the lactate threshold higher*, so that they can stay in a zone where they burn a higher percentage of fat, even though they are at a pretty high percent of their max. And as long as they stay below that now-higher lactate threshold, they will burn a ton of fat and *never hit The Wall.*

Moving the Lactate Threshold

An obese, out-of-shape person hits the lactate threshold at about 50 percent of his max or even less. That's why people in awful shape can barely walk up a flight of stairs without getting winded. Someone who is trained can move that threshold up to 60 to 70 percent of max. People who work out a lot often have a threshold in the low 80 percent range. Hell, my lactate threshold is 80 percent and I'm not an endurance athlete. We are able to keep on going *indefinitely* at a pretty fast clip. And of course, burn more fat the whole time. It is a win-win.

There's more. In the normal course, glucose or glycogen (different forms of sugar) are much, much easier to access than fat. And the body turns to them first (but not exclusively) and stays with them, for much of its fuel, for a long time. But when you get in good shape, your body learns to *access fat sooner*. The body learns to go for belly fat much earlier and thus helps you lose that ugly (and dangerous) stuff much earlier.

Another one: Fit people's hearts work better. A fit, heavily exercised heart is a stronger muscle, and it moves a larger volume of blood with each beat. The little engines (mitochondria) get more fuel and go faster and longer.

Finally, fit people also have more of the enzymes that reach out and grab free fat in the blood. These little guys are like Pac Men: They chomp into free fat (in the bloodstream and elsewhere) and make it usable by the muscles as fuel, much earlier in the game. In other words, fitness brings all kinds of miracles, all of them good.

All You Really Need to Know Is . . .

O kay, we're done. And there will not be a quiz. All you need to take away from this complex chapter is this: *Doing hard exercise like serious intervals* on alternate days moves your lactate threshold up, which makes you more fit. That means that you can go faster and keep it up longer. You look and feel better. All of which is terrific.

Final reminder: Doing any aerobic exercise, four days a week, is a triumph. Healthy is wonderful. Healthy and fit . . . well, it's quite a lot more.

CHAPTER SIX

The Astonishing Importance of Strength Training

A recent study began with the grim statement that, in the normal course, people lose 10 percent of their muscle mass per decade after age forty. And that it gets worse after seventy. You lose muscle mass and suffer a serious accretion of fat into the muscles. But here's the great news: They took a look at cadres of serious athletes in their forties, up to their eighties. The muscle loss didn't happen to them. The seventy- and eighty-year-old athletes had about as much muscle mass as the athletes in their forties. There was some drop-off at age fifty, but not much. And there was little further decline after that. Other studies support the same conclusion. That, kids, is amazingly good news.

Is strength training hellish for many of us? You bet. Is it worth it? Oh, yes!

That was a study of serious lifelong athletes. Will it work if you're starting later in life? Less clear, but yes. What studies there are say it certainly will. So there you sit, asking uneasily if you are really supposed to toddle off to the gym two or three times a week in costumes that do not flatter and pick up heavy metal or use nasty machines till you drop. And the answer is, "Umm, yeah, you are."

Quality of Life: Four Amazing Things Strength Training Does for You

Aerobic exercise does more to stop death, but strength training makes living worthwhile.

—Dr. Henry Lodge

et me talk for a minute about the miraculous "quality of life" reasons for strength training. There were five amazing things that aerobics did for you. Strength training is almost as important and, sure enough, there are four amazing things it does for you, which you should know about.

1. Strength training makes you stronger. Duh! But it does, and it does it remarkably fast. And that is more important than you might think. You can have a 35 to 50 percent increase in strength in just six months. And that makes such a difference. Not just to get out of the chair, climb the stairs, all that, but to avoid falling. Falls are one of the great interrupters of life, after fifty or sixty—the Third Act. The curtain comes down, and it may not go back up. Not on the same play, anyhow. After age fifty, a fall can alter your life. Maybe end it. Hard to believe when you're young, but true.

And there are few things as important as plain strength, especially strength in your legs, to prevent falls and keep you mobile in general. In the absence of serious strength training you will lose some 10 percent of your strength each decade after age forty; that's the default-to-decay business at work. You have to send grow messages over that signaling system, kids, to avoid that muscle loss. You have to overcome that tide. Few things matter as much as simply avoiding sarcopenia (the loss of muscle mass and muscle signaling with age) and you do that best with strength training.

2. Strength training grows new bone. One of the worst things about the tide of aging is that it is sucking the bone out of your bones. All of us lose bone mass at the rate of up to 1 percent a year. Women, during and after menopause, lose bone mass at the rate of up to 2 percent a year, with terrifying results. By the age of sixty, a woman will have lost up to 30 percent of all the bone she ever had to see her through her long life. And you have no idea this is happening to you, because osteoporosis is a silent disease. Listen to these numbers: A woman falls down after age sixty and has the traditional older woman's injury, a broken hip. Fifty percent of the women who have that break will never walk unaided again: It is the cane, the walker, and the chair. And 20 percent will be dead

---

THE DOCTOR IS IN: Osteoporosis

Osteoporosis kills more women than breast cancer. But here's what you have to remember: Osteoporosis is optional. All you have to do to avoid this epidemic of broken bones and broken lives is (1) keep your bones strong and (2) don't fall down. Lifting weights is the single best thing you can do to turn the tide of losing bone mass and preventing falls.

within one year. Those are appalling numbers. And it is all because of osteoporosis, silent bone loss with aging.

The only thing that stops or slows bone loss is serious, consistent strength training. Calcium with vitamin D helps a little, but it doesn't help much. Aerobics is not enough; it doesn't put enough stress on the bones to stimulate them to grow. The only real answer is serious strength training.

3. Strength training renews and strengthens your internal signaling system and restores balance and coordination. In the normal course of aging you lose balance, proprioception (the sense of where you are in space), and coordination at the rate of some 12 percent a decade—much like muscle mass. And it is brutal. The cumulative effect threatens to make you into a ridiculous stumbling old man, an absurdly fragile old woman. Not the star of your own glorious Third Act.

Balance is so important, and you can radically improve it with strength training. Do it right, the way we'll teach, and you can have pretty good balance, for most of the rest of your life.

4. Strength training relieves pain. It is the great anodyne, the reliever of pain that is already here, and the armor against pain to come. It is not perfect. Pain will come with age. But strength training does more than anything else to hold it at bay. You will not know until you get there, but pain is the great handmaiden of aging, and it is a curse. A relatively little bit of chronic pain soaks up your attention and cuts you off from others. It slows you way down. It makes you walk funny. You want to talk about it all the time, which is a real curse. For everyone. It transports you into the land of the fragile old.

Good strength training will do more than anything else to fight

---

THE DOCTOR IS IN: The Good Stress of
Weight Training

Remember what you learned earlier about C-6 and C-10 back
in Chapter One? Well, the motions of daily life are not enough
to turn on the C-10 of growth. It takes a critical amount of effort to
cross that threshold and secrete enough C-6 to trigger the production
of C-10. You get this through strength training. You need to do
strength training to cross that threshold for power and coordination,
to get C-10 into your neural networks, into the meat of your muscles,
into your joints, and into your tendons.

Aerobic exercise takes you across the threshold for endurance,
circulation, and longevity, but you need strength training for power
and neural coordination. A single step on level ground doesn't turn
on C-10. Nor does climbing a few stairs. But climbing stairs until
you feel your legs burn will turn on C-10. Lifting weights until you
can't lift them anymore? That really turns on C-10.

This is why you have to push to the point of muscle fatigue with
weights—to that burning feeling in your muscles that most of us
would skip if we could. A trainer (see page 68) will eventually make
sure you lift enough weight to cycle all the way through the reserve
capacity of your strength cells. To lift ten or twelve times in a row
and then do it again. Done right, you will drain your muscles of all
their energy and then force them to contract a few more times. That's
the critical part; that's how you intentionally damage your muscle
cells. Not your muscles, just the muscle cells. And you damage them
quite a lot. On purpose. Electron microscope pictures of muscle
show extensive damage at the cellular level after a weight workout.
That's fine and what your body needs. Your muscles will quiver and
burn, which is not fun, but inside you will be forcing your brain to
activate all your strength units. Do this for three sets, and you will
have forced your body to damage all those strength units, which then
forces it to repair all those strength units. Growth, strength—youth.

(By the way, don't confuse damaging your muscle cells
by exhausting them with damaging your muscles and joints by
overloading them.)

off and reverse chronic pain—arthritis, bursitis, sore joints of all kinds—and your wretched sore back.

Hire a Trainer

The first thing to do as you embark on a strength-training regimen is to read this book—all of it. I mean it: Don't just read the beginning and jump in. It is also a great idea to get Bill Fabrocini's DVDs (see page 121), which are invaluable in getting you started and keeping you on the proper path. For some, hiring a trainer is also a good idea.

Trainers are expensive, lord knows, but they can be worth it, at least to begin with. You'll have fewer injuries and a more efficient workout. This is a lifelong commitment, after all, and why not get your posture, alignment, core strength, and "muscle memory" right from the get-go? A good trainer can help you to do the exercises correctly. He or she will teach you what weights to use, and when and by what increments to increase them. Even more important, a good one can motivate you and keep you going, like nothing else. That will help.

How do you find a good one? That, I am afraid, is a bit murky. There are various accrediting agencies such as the American Council on Exercise, the American College of Sports Medicine, and the National Academy of Sports Medicine, among others. Ask your gym about what trainers they'd recommend. When talking to potential trainers, ask how they feel about machines versus techniques that use your own weight and how they feel about the importance of "isolating" muscles for training. If he or she is keen on that, that person is more of a bodybuilder and may not be the trainer for you. Find somebody sympathetic but someone who will also push you.

THE DOCTOR IS IN: Arthritis Is No Excuse

People with arthritis often see it as a barrier to strength training. But arthritis is rarely a contraindication. Quite the contrary. The combination of strong muscles and improved proprioception protects the joints from further damage and lets them heal. Most arthritis patients report about a 50 percent reduction in pain and limitation with several months of strength training; minor arthritis usually disappears entirely. All those aches and pains do make it trickier to get started, however, particularly if you have significant arthritis. If that describes you, talk to your doctor about having a physical therapist guide you in the initial stages of your weight-training program. If the arthritis is in your hands, ask a physical therapist about strength exercises for your hands. But unless your doctor tells you to stop, never let arthritis keep you from exercising. There are a few exceptions to this, but for everyone else, remember that arthritis is an inflammatory condition. It's a disease of C-6, so treat it with C-10.

Some patients tell me they can't do weights because they have arthritis and it hurts. Think about this: For most forms of arthritis, the prescription is a six-week course of physical therapy. But physical therapy is mostly just six weeks of supervised weight training. Six weeks because your insurance coverage runs out after that. But you shouldn't be doing it for six weeks; you should be doing it for life, two times a week. That's how to prevent most forms of arthritis if you don't already have it. And to make it better if you do.

We Live in Glass Boxes

Years ago, Bill was struggling to explain to me what he felt so strongly about: the enormous importance of compound, whole-body movement. It was in the early days, and his message wasn't sinking in.

Look, he said, we all live in glass boxes. And their size and shape are defined by our ability to move—our balance, our range of motion, the soundness of our joints and muscles, our proprioception and coordination—all those things. He balanced himself, his feet well apart, and moved as he talked. He moves constantly when he talks about this stuff because he is so into it.

He twisted his hips sharply from side to side—reached out to the sides with his hands, toward the back, out toward me, over his head. It's not having powerful biceps or quads or whatever that matters in the end, he said. It's how well they work together with your signaling system and the little muscles and joints to reach out. Which he did. And up. And he reached way down to touch the floor, outside his right foot, and way up over his head and to the left with his hands, stretching as high as he could.

He went on for a while, and it began to resonate: We live in these glass boxes, all of us, all our lives. And they set the outer limits of our ability to move: from side to side, and back and forth, and up and down. Range of motion, flexibility, sound joints. As we get older and lose balance, strength, and mobility—as our joints go—the glass boxes get smaller. When we are very old, the box tends to get very small indeed. Not much bigger than a coffin really, one of those old wooden jobs, without much elbow room.

Do nothing, and that glass box starts to shrink in your thirties. And by the time you are sixty, it can be pretty tight. The quality of your life has everything to do with the size of your glass box, and it can get awfully darn small.

But it doesn't have to. To a surprising extent, the size of your glass box, all the way through life, is in your own control. Balance is trainable. Proprioception is trainable. Coordination is trainable. Strength is trainable. Fundamentally, the whole signaling system and the combination of signals, small and large muscles, and ligaments can be refreshed and strengthened by the right kind of strength training.

To get a better sense of it, Bill says, think of a great skier— Bode Miller, for example. Look at him during a race. He is cantilevered way out to one side, almost touching the snow, as he goes screaming around a gate at sixty miles an hour over a rutted icy surface. The next gate comes up in a heartbeat. With amazing force, he swings up and over to the other side. Boom! All those horrendous g-forces, still at sixty miles an hour, screaming down the hill but on the other side now. Different muscles, different joints, different cascades of signals. And still canted out so far to the other side, he almost touches the snow. He flips back and forth like this again and again in a single race while making astonishing microadjustments in the angle of his feet, the degree of lean, the cant of his hips, so that he is faster at this than anyone else in the world. He has a huge glass box. And he does exercises all the time to preserve it.

None of us ever had a glass box like Bode Miller's. Too bad. But the important point is that we can preserve and extend our glass box enormously, with the right exercises. In many of the exercises you are going to do, you will be stretching your glass box as if it were made of plastic wrap, not glass, and you could literally push it out and make it bigger. It can be done, no matter how old you are, no matter the size of your glass box. And it's a great idea.

CHAPTER SEVEN

Train Movements, Not Muscles: Whole-Body Movement

Modern strength training grew out of the old model of the bodybuilding movement of the 1960s and 1970s when Arnold Schwarzenegger and the movie *Pumping Iron* were all the rage. But it also grew out of the development of modern weight-training machines. The Nautilus machine was a brilliant invention by a genius named Arthur Jones that used complex cams and pulleys to maintain even pressure on muscles throughout a given exercise. And significantly, it promoted muscle stress over a "full range of motion." The new Nautilus machines—and their progeny and competitors—were great gadgets, and they pulled people into gyms. Partly because they were kind of fun, partly because they were more or less safe, and partly because they were easy to use. And they did build muscle, as millions know. Anyhow, Nautilus and its rivals and successors have been at the heart of the conditioning movement for the last forty years. You see them, wall-to-wall, in every gym in the country.

Posture, Stability, Movement: The New Model

But there were problems. Problems with the machines, and serious problems with using bodybuilding as a model for strength training. Bodybuilders are wonderful looking, if that's your taste (not mine, I confess), but their bodies don't work very well. They don't move very well. And they don't last well over time. You'd think we would have focused on that over all those years of using the machines. But somehow we didn't.

Bill Fabrocini tells this interesting story about a client who had been a great success in life and who had been very serious about his weight-lifting regimen. At seventy he was built like a bull with bulging muscles, and he could bench-press almost three hundred pounds. Trouble was, he was falling apart. Hideous back pain, horrible shoulder joints, awful knees and hips, everything. He couldn't sleep for the pain. What had happened, Bill said, was that decades of isolating and lifting had worn away his joints and ruined his posture. He couldn't move normally and his balance was atrocious. When you took the support of the bench away, he was really weak. His coordination was terrible, and he struggled to lift anything that required whole-body movement, which is most things. And he was looking at serious neck and other joint surgeries.

Bill took him under his wing. It took a while—two years. Two years of emphasis on the joints and Bill's philosophy of whole-body movement. But in time the client's joints stopped hurting, his posture improved radically, and he could move freely. The doctor who had been discussing surgery was shocked and delighted at the changes. Today, surgery is off the table, he is stronger than ever—stronger in motion—and he does not hurt. Happy guy. He ought to be.

That is an isolated anecdote, but it makes profound sense because of the bodybuilder's focus on muscles, not movement. As far as Bill (and this book) is concerned, movement is the whole point. We train to move, not to strike poses for the cover of *Men's Health* or the judges in the Mr. Peoria contest. And that leads to Bill's fundamental point: Train movements, not muscles. This is a concept shared by all the best trainers and fitness people in the country.

But today's great revolution is mostly a revolution away from machines. You do not have to get over machines, and you certainly do not have to drop them completely from your strength-training regimen. But you should know about the alternatives, the much better alternatives, and what's so good about them.

The miracle of the new strength training is complex adaptation to movement. Training creates muscular and—even more important—signaling adaptations to improve movement. You literally tear down and rebuild the muscle cells and rewire the neurotransmitters that control them. That's how you adapt. That's how you avoid the tide of aging. In this book, we are training you for life. Your life. For a life of lifting stuff off a shelf, riding a bike, getting out of a chair, walking to work, paddling a kayak, picking up a kid, hitting a hell of a golf drive. Training for life. A long one. It sounds a bit doctrinaire and bookish when you first hear it, but don't worry, it makes profound sense. And it will sink in. Give us a few pages.

Life and Movement
in Three Dimensions

Life is movement, and movement is very different from muscle-isolation training, the kind of training you get on most machines. The focus of machines and bodybuilding is on isolating and building specific muscles. You sit down at the bicep curl machine, you put your elbows on the pad, and away you go: You isolate and strengthen your biceps. But movement does not involve muscles in isolation and a single plane. It involves muscles—and bones and sinews and the amazing signaling system—working in elaborate concert, in three dimensions and three planes, in depth.

Think about any athletic move—a tennis serve or a golf drive, for example. Your arms and hands do the last bits, but tennis and golf are not hand and arm sports. They are whole-body sports, like just about everything else.

All the power, for example, comes roaring up from the great muscles in your legs, then from the fierce torquing of your whole body, and only toward the end is it your shoulders, arms, and hands. The effectiveness is mostly a matter of transmitting and enhancing that power through the core. Transmitting it—with the least loss or "spill"—up to the shoulders and beyond. Golf is a whole-body exercise. Skiing is a whole-body exercise. Living is a whole-body exercise—a compound, complex exercise in three dimensions, often involving significant rotation. If you are training for sports, or for life, you are training for complex movement. If you are training for complex movement, do complex movement. Which mostly means using free weights or your body, elastic tubes, or machines that put a premium on balance and whole-body coordination.

Free weights are better for you than machines because they involve balancing and subtle corrections from side to side, all of which use and strengthen a whole bunch of other muscles and neuro-connectors that are at the heart of your ability to function well in the real world. It's not just strength that matters; it's the wiring, too. But I recognize that doing free weights takes some getting used to, and they are harder than using machines. So, for heaven's sake, do not drop machines if doing so is going to keep you from doing strength training at all. That would be the worst possible result. But it is our hope that you will try working at the free-weight, whole-body approach that Bill will teach you here. It is better for you.

One of the great things about whole-body exercises is that they are terrific for training and developing your balance. A great flaw in the machines—and the reason they are easy to use—is that they do the balancing for you. You don't learn how, and you don't develop the networks of muscles and signals that make balance possible. Squats and lunges are hard because you have to balance. But here's the deal: Balance is trainable. You can improve it radically, at any age, by doing exercises that require balance. Bill gives you one-legged exercises in Chapter Nine, and many of his strength-training exercises require, and so improve, your balance.

Signaling in Three Dimensions

Think for a second about the signaling system that supports all movement. As you now know better than most people in the gym, the body's signaling system is the key to movement. Every muscle fiber—in addition to every cell—has its own neuro-connector that tells it when to fire, the sequencing that is the key to coordination, to everything. There are billions of them. And those signals are coordinated body-wide. It's one grid. The integration of those billions of signals is of the essence. It is what movement

THE DOCTOR IS IN: Signaling

Whole-body training is important because it makes your body smarter as well as stronger. This gets us into signaling, and strength and balance training are your tools for staying nimble, agile, and vital for the years ahead.

Strength training works on those signals that control proprioception (the sense of where your body is in space), coordination, and balance. Pushing a muscle hard sends a blaring signal back up to the brain. Remember the instant tightening of your joints as you start to climb stairs? This is important stuff for your body. If your brain slacks off for an instant, and you don't make the split-second adjustments, you might pull a muscle or sprain an ankle. So the signals to your brain from strength training are loud and important—priority news. And they create growth— first in the signaling pathways themselves, blazing that direct trail through the forest of neural networks, and second in the muscles, tendons, ligaments, and joints directly. With this growth comes a new integration between your brain and body. They have always been fused; we just forgot it. This is how you reconnect them. It's a literal, physical reconnection: nerve fibers you can see under the microscope, brain chemistry you can see on MRI scans, reaction time you can measure in the lab. It's skiing better, feeling stronger, feeling better.

is all about. So start with this: Strength training is signal training. Not one signal at a time, either. Or even a million at a time—all of them. They work together; that's the deal.

And this science has some strong implications for how you train. You train for integrated, instinctive movement. You cannot make up your conscious mind to move a muscle cell and do it. It doesn't work that way. Ultimately, it is a matter of muscle-group memory. Of remembering and recruiting the movement, not the

Chris's Bum Hip

L et me give you an example from life that has been curiously underreported in the popular press: the gripping story of my bum hip. I had been a good kid about exercise, having spent zillions of hours on my bike and done a lot of old-fashioned weight lifting, especially on leg-press machines. It worked in the sense that my legs were very strong. I can leg press four hundred pounds all afternoon. But here's the funny thing. The muscles like the psoas and the gluteus maximus that support the hip and the signals that run through them—those muscles were not being worked enough, or correctly. And sure enough, they rotted. Just a little bit. Just enough so that my hip joint got a teeny bit out of alignment. And slowly, slowly, over time, things started to chew on themselves in there. And one day, on a strange squat machine, I tore my labrum (a cartilage cuff that helps hold the hip joint in place).

That's the mishap Bill eventually diagnosed and that was fixed in an operation. The operation involved a lot of pain and expense and rehab. The hip is much better but still not perfect. It never will be. All of which I might have avoided if I had done more whole-body exercise. Like free-standing squats and lunges, to look after the support muscles and the wiring.

muscles. It is a whole-body affair. Strength per se is relatively minor. You want strength and you must have it; you surely must have substantial lean muscle mass. But signaling comes first. Signaling actually *is* strength to a remarkable extent. You can beef up the raw power of the cells, but signals come first, always.

And signals work on a whole-body basis. The power grid of the body is an integrated one, or we could not move the way we do. That is what grace and coordination are all about—the well-tempered signaling system of the whole body. Bill's basic point begins to be obvious: We do not live in a two-dimensional world. Ever. And our muscles do not work in isolation. Ever. We use our muscles in concert, and only in concert.

Concert is a good word for it, as a matter of fact. Muscle movement is music. And it is not solo music. Not a bicep solo or a quad solo. It is a concert every time. Bode Miller screams around a gate on skis; he uses every muscle in his body in concert. Train the orchestra, not just the bassoons. Do the bassoons get a little separate training once in a while? Sure. And the violins and the drums? Of course. So use the isolation machines occasionally to strengthen certain muscles. But remember it is an orchestra you are running here. Train the orchestra.

Compound, whole-body exercise makes sense for a bunch of reasons, but one of them is particularly important if you happen to be over forty. Or seventy. Remember the warning from earlier in the book that the stuff you don't use rots? Muscles that are not used rot. Sinews that are not used rot. And most important of all, signaling systems that are not used rot. You can use machines that isolate and strengthen some muscles all day long, and rot can still be going on in the supporting muscles (and signaling systems) that are being carefully excluded from the exercise. Well, the poor little guys who get excluded have their revenge. They rot. And when they do, they take down the big boys, too.

Boomers and the Shrinking Margin for Error

The advice in this book—and the exercises—will work like a charm for everyone, whether twenty or sixty. They are as close to universal as we can make them. But the advice and the exercises are much more important for men and women who are no longer twenty or thirty-five. They are hugely important for boomers and beyond.

Think about a couple of things. Your prospects now, your upside, are greater than you had dared to dream. Much greater than they were when you were twenty. True. But it is also true that you are not twenty anymore. And there are consequences. A lot of you, as many as 80 percent, have had some loss of mobility: a bum hip, a bum shoulder, a bum knee. Some pain, some loss of flex-ibility. And you are a bit more vulnerable. Your "margin for error in movement" has shrunk a little. Work out more, not less, and you will improve the margins. But do it wisely. Because the margin for error is narrower.

After forty, doing strength training right matters more and more. Doing it at all matters most, of course. That is the great key to a good Third Act. But you are not bulletproof. When you were a kid—like most of the trainers in most of the gyms—you could jump on any machine without warming up and bang out however many reps and be fine. And you could use them any old way. Form mattered less because you had such a huge margin for error. Today, it is more important to warm up, the right way. The right technique is critical. It is more important to set your core before you lift. It is more important to rotate your hips, not your lower back. The margins for error have shrunk. The cost of doing things wrong has gone up. Much of our focus in Chapter Ten is on doing strength training correctly, so you can keep on moving forever. And not get hurt.

CHAPTER EIGHT

The Three Little Pigs, or Posture and a Strong Core

All right, now let's talk about something that may strike you as a bit dull but is *really, really* important. As important as anything in the book, as a matter of fact. Let's talk about posture and the core.

Actually, let's not do that yet. They are so scary sounding; one hears one's mother's voice. Or the junior high school gym teacher. Instead, let's talk for a minute about "The Three Little Pigs."

You will perhaps recall the heartbreaking story of the three little pigs and the Big Bad Wolf. Two of the little pigs—the two fun ones, it always seemed to me—slapped together crappy houses out of straw and twigs. Didn't take any time at all, and they were delighted with themselves and their shoddy houses. But sure enough, the Big Bad Wolf came around and simply blew 'em down, and ate the two nice pigs. Awful.

The third little pig—who always struck me as a bit pompous—had warned his brothers, but to no avail. So he went off and—with great care—built his house out of brick. The Big Bad Wolf showed up and made ugly threats, which the third little pig was pleased to ignore. And then the wolf huffed and puffed—no luck. This house was strong and the wolf was screwed. He eventually had to go off to McDonald's or something. Ate crap and died. The third little pig, the smug and sanctimonious one, lived to be ninety-five, was married three times, and had 1,037 piglets (he was a pig, after all). I hate to use the smug little pig to illustrate a moral, but I have no choice. He was absolutely right.

You will be relieved to learn that I tell this ancient nursery story for a reason. Turns out, there is a Big Bad Wolf in all of our lives. And about 80 percent of us—maybe 90—live in straw or stick houses. Not a good idea in a wolf-infested neighborhood like ours. Mercifully, the wolf does not actually eat us anymore. But he does cause little problems. For example, let me ask you this: Does your back hurt?

Of course, your back hurts, you dope! I do not mean to sound smug, like that third little pig, but of course your back hurts. Your back hurts like crazy because you live in a house that is a dangerous, tilted wreck, slapped together out of sticks and straw. Your posture stinks; you don't even know the terms stacking *or* alignment. *Your core is weak so you leak energy at every step. You don't know how to move—or lift or twist or crouch—so you're doomed to a life of serious back pain that is only going to get worse. The wolf is contentedly gnawing on your backbone. And he will not stop until you rebuild your damned house. Straight and aligned, brick by brick. With a solid core.* Pills won't help. There are no guarantees with back surgery either. You gotta rebuild the house. Even if you wind up needing surgery you *still* have to rebuild the house sooner or later. Better to do it sooner.

The pleasing news is that Bill Fabrocini—who has been such a help to me and thousands of others—is going to show you how. It is not going to be easy, and it will take a lot of change. But it will work and be worth it—a bit technical in places but very important. Because the junk pile you live in now, well, it just isn't safe.

What Is Good Posture?

Building a good brick house is a three-step process. The first one is architecture, structure. You have to get the walls and the support beams in place. And they have to be straight. For you, that means good posture. You have to *stand up straight.*

Bill says that there are forces at work on our body much like the geological forces in nature, so we have to expect a certain amount of wear and tear. There's basic gravity, which means things begin to drift/slope downward, and there are all the twisting, compression, and shear forces we generate in daily life. Bending, lifting, and twisting a few million times intensifies the influence of those forces on our bodies. They don't amount to that much on a given day or over a year. But over a lifetime, they can have profound consequences. They can turn your backbone into rubble.

And of course, there is aging. As we get older, physical habits (sitting at a computer or slumping on the den couch) cause some muscles to tighten and others to become weak, pulling our bones out of their natural alignment. And this is made much worse if we do not pay attention to and take decent care of our bodies. The original sin of bad self-care is bad posture. Rotten posture opens the door for the Big Bad Wolf. Rotten posture—and especially rotten posture in motion—brings us low.

Good posture is the key to muscle and joint alignment. If it is not natural to you, achieving good posture is a bit dodgy. The great trick is to have what's called a neutral spine. And to have your body properly stacked. What in the world does that mean?

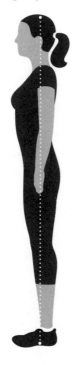

To get an idea, look at the picture at the left. See the gentle curves of her back: That's perfect. It's what is called a neutral spine. See the very slight arch of her lower, or lumbar, spine? That's the key part. You don't want to be hunched over, which eliminates or flattens out that curve. You certainly don't want to be swaybacked, which exaggerates that curve and thrusts out your butt. And you don't want your head jutting forward. You want to be just right. Her shoulders are back and down, chin neither lifting or tucking, ears directly over the shoulders, weight straight up and down on the hips, knees, and feet. When you have it right, you should be able to draw a plumb line straight down through your ear, shoulder, hip, knee, and ankle. That's what's called alignment. If you have a trainer, get him or her to drill you on posture.

Getting this right is a game changer in your life, and it is critical before embarking on a weight-training program. So spend some time on it. Look at yourself in a full-length mirror—from both the front and the side. Take a good look at the way you stand naturally: Are your shoulders hunched around your ears? Is one shoulder higher than the other? Is your back rounded? Does your head jut forward? Do you have more weight on one leg than the other? Is your chest collapsed or lifted? What about your stomach—are your abdominal muscles contracted? Are your front ribs splayed out in an effort to overcorrect? Now, don't go all negative on yourself. We all get into bad habits. And we can change.

Once you've done this assessment, shake yourself all over, loosen up, and take some deep breaths. Now go back to the mirror. Start with your weight distributed evenly on your feet. Roll your shoulders gently back and down, away from your ears. You have no business putting your shoulders in your ears; that is *wrong, Sir*! Suck in your gut. Get your head back. Now turn your body to the side and check to see if your ears, shoulders, hips, knees, and ankles are aligned. Remember that plumb line going down through the crown of your head to your feet?

Key, key point. Bad posture is always bad. But having bad posture when you are exercising—and especially when you are doing strength training—is a dangerous horror. Honest. It is terribly important that you do all Bill's movements with a neutral spine (that means keeping that slight arch in the lower back) and with your body in alignment. Bill reminds you here and your trainer will remind you in the gym. You must *set your posture* before each exercise. And tighten your core. (It is mostly a matter of contracting your abs, as if someone were about to tap you in the gut.) Check on both throughout a given exercise. If your back starts rounding, for example, something's wrong. Stop. Adjust and go on. Make yourself think about good posture all the time, until the glorious day when it becomes your natural posture, and when tightening your core becomes a natural part of beginning any exercise. That day *will* come. Honest.

A Note About Sitting

Sitting, it turns out, is full of dark perils (groan). First, we do too much of it. It is a superb idea to get up and move around. Every fifteen minutes, say. Indeed, any movement, including small movement, is a great idea. Oh, and here is some more dreary news: Even when you are sitting, remember your posture—keep your feet on the floor and knees aligned over ankles, your spine neutral. And get out of the habit of crossing your knees—it pulls the spine out of alignment. I do it once in a while just for the hell of it. But I am bad.

What's Wrong with This Picture?

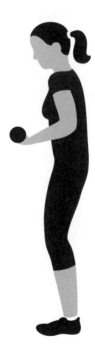

Maybe the clearest way to demonstrate what we mean about posture is to show you what happens when you ignore good posture or don't have enough core stability. Look at the picture of the woman (right) with her shoulders hunched and her head forward. Very common mistakes. Your head, with good posture (not slouched forward), weighs about twelve pounds on your neck and spine. When you slouch: thirty-seven pounds. That is quite the extra load, all on your neck and spine. It is, for

Bill Says: *Exercising with bad posture and a weak or unengaged core can be much, much worse than not exercising at all.*

sure, the difference between a healthy neck and spine and a badly tortured one. I am not your mother but *stand up straight. And keep your head back.* If you don't know what we mean by "keep your head back," think of a turtle, retracting its head into its shell. Bill says, pull your head back like a turtle pulling into his shell. You'll both be safer that way.

I suspect this is all obvious by now, but let me just wail on you for a moment longer and try to scare you. If you slouch and let your shoulders fall forward and let your lower back go flat, you put much more pressure on your lower, or lumbar, spine. And that is where almost all back pain begins. Not just the pain either—bad backs, with operations and stuff. And it is much worse if you slump when you lift weights, as this poor creature is doing. You put horrendous pressure on the front of the disks. Eventually, you are going to squeeze the resilience out of the disks and flatten them on one side so they can't do their job. And in the long term, you are going to tear a disk, the dreaded ruptured disk, and it means serious trouble. When someone with Bill's eye (or even mine) walks through a gym, we see dozens of people like this. Don't let that be you.

Do Not Bend, Lift, and Twist with Your Back

Y ou should know that your lower back, your lumbar spine, is not designed to rotate. If you learn nothing else in these exercise chapters, learn this: *Do not bend, lift, and twist at the same time with your spine. Lots of compound motions are great; this one is disastrous.*

Your upper and middle back can do some rotating, but—even if you are mostly using your upper back—the bend-lift-twist move from your back is not a good idea. It is inevitable that you will bend, lift, and twist in any good exercise regimen. But the great trick is: *Always rotate with your hips, not your back.* Lower back rotation with weight is suicidal. Here is the mantra one more time: *Do not bend, lift, and twist with your back!* Ever. It will make a mess. *Rotate with your hips.*

Stability and a Strong Core

Your spine, a miraculously powerful but flexible structure, is made up of a stack of bones (the vertebrae), intermediate washers or shock absorbers made of spongelike gristle (disks), and a bunch of wires (sinews). And a powerful network of muscles and fascia tissue. The whole business—everything but your arms, legs, and head—is your core. It is an elaborate structure and works remarkably well. But it is not bulletproof. About 80 percent of the people in this country have back pain bad enough to have sought medical help.

Your back is designed to tolerate remarkable loads when it is aligned properly, that is, when you have good posture. You have to stand up straight. You have to sit up straight. And you have to develop a strong core.

The second leg of Bill's stool, after posture, is stability. Stability is having your core, or the girdle of muscles that holds your back steady, strong and engaged. Engaging or activating it is a simple matter of tensing your core muscles slightly. People tend to think of the core as just the abs, the so-called six-pack you see on the covers of magazines. It is a lot more than that. In fact, it is a set of several overlapping bands of muscles that run from your front to your back and all the way up to your neck. The upper abs are just one—and a rather minor one—out of a bunch. You need your whole core to be strong. The warm-up exercises in Chapter Nine are heavily focused on doing just that. And many of the Twenty-Five Sacred Exercises emphasize the strengthening and engagement of the core. Certainly the crunches, and the planks, as well as the squats and lunges. And my favorite, Number 13, the chop with the medicine ball. A strong core stabilizes your spine, keeps your body in alignment, and improves your posture. Getting a grip on your abdominals and the low back muscles are key to relieving lower back pain. You must have a strong core so you can move with safety and power.

A Word for Athletes

A properly stacked body—a body with a neutral spine and a solid, engaged core—is more resilient so it can tolerate up to 40 percent more load than one with bad posture. Good athletes have good posture because it works. And good athletes work hard at their core strength, which is the bedrock of good posture. Tiger Woods had his problems but not with his core. He spent thousands of hours doing core exercises. He is famous for it. Want to be a better golfer? Strengthen your core. Want to be skiing downhill in your eighties? Strengthen your core. Want to be on your feet and not on a walker or in a chair, all the way to the waterfall? Strengthen your core. And watch your posture. It will see you through.

The goal of Bill's PSM (Posture, Stability, and Movement) is successful movement, in three dimensions, with force, and without getting hurt. It is a matter of having good posture supported by good core strength and stability. On to Preparation for Movement, or warming up.

CHAPTER NINE

Preparation for Movement: The Warm-Ups

Bill Fabrocini calls his warm-up regimen "preparation for movement." He does it himself, every single day, no joke—I've seen it. Because he knows—from thousands of hours spent looking at men and women who have made a hash of their joints—how important it is. This is a whole-body warm-up but with special emphasis on the joints. It does the traditional and important business of warming up the blood and the muscles and so on, but the focus is on the joints. On your hips. And your poor back. And your ankles. Oh, and your knees. Do please remember that 80 percent of the people in this country have impaired movement in their hips and bad backs. The difficulty frequently starts with the hips or ankles. And guess what? These unpleasant phenomena are closely related. Step 1 on the road to *preventing or reversing* loss of hip mobility—or ankle mobility or shoulder mobility—is this set of "preparations for movement."

The first time, the warm-up alone may take a half hour or more. Who cares—you're learning. I now do them in about ten minutes, as does Bill. If it takes you longer, even after you've been at it for a while, then take fifteen minutes—but don't skip them. Find your own way.

Each exercise starts with the challenge, "Why Bother?" which pinpoints the focus of the warm-up and why it is good for you. If you understand the "why" of the movement, it sticks. The step-by-step instructions that follow are accompanied by annotated illustrations. The "Bill Says" are special tips based on years of Bill's experience training thousands of clients. They are meant to act as a checkpoint to help you avoid bad habits and common pitfalls. It's like having a trainer right beside you.

General Rules

Here are some general rules for all of these warm-up exercises:

1. Do ten reps of each exercise, unless fewer are specified.

2. Move at a slow to moderate speed (except for the footwork pieces).

3. Do these "pain free" other than some discomfort from the stretch in a few exercises. A little muscle pain is okay— joint pain is not.

4. Slowly increase the range of motion for each exercise with each repetition.

When you are told to contract your abs (abdominal muscles) or glutes (gluteal muscles), use light to moderate force. Be gentle yet focused on these muscles. Think about the muscles involved. Visualize what you're doing. Be sure that you are breathing throughout each exercise and not focusing so hard that you're holding your breath.

Equipment

The only equipment needed for the warm-ups is a mat and either a bench or a chair. The warm-ups go in this order: (1) Start on your back; (2) Roll over on your stomach; (3) Roll up on your side (both sides); (4) Get up on all fours; (5) Kneeling; (6) Stand up. This will help you remember.

> Download a six-page illustrated cheat sheet
> for the Warm-Ups at youngernextyear.com.

ON YOUR BACK

The Bridge

Why Bother? This exercise is designed to loosen and warm up your joints, in this case your hips. It's especially good for your glutes, which are your dominant hip extensors. This is a critical muscle that weakens with aging, reducing hip mobility. The Bridge also works on your core and lower back.

Step 1: Lie on your back with both legs bent, your heels almost directly under your knees. Push through your heels and lift your butt off the floor. Tighten your abs and squeeze your glutes. Hold for five seconds.

Step 2: Slowly roll down through your spine. Repeat.

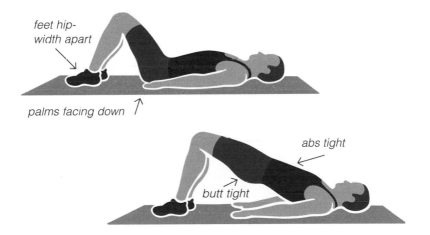

feet hip-width apart

palms facing down

abs tight

butt tight

Bill Says: *If you like, put a ball or block between your thighs and squeeze it as you go up into the Bridge. It gets the glutes more involved.*

WARM-UPS

Leg Raise

Why Bother? This one is good to get the hip flexors and core activated, and to lengthen the hamstrings and calf muscles.

Step 1: Lie on your back, with one knee bent, foot on the floor, and the other leg straight. Contract your abs. Tense the quad and flex the foot of the straight leg, then lift it upward, flexing at the hip until you feel a hamstring or calf stretch. Like a rubber band, it will "recoil" your leg back to the floor. When kicking leg up, lower back must stay still.

Step 2: Do ten lifts, then switch sides and repeat.

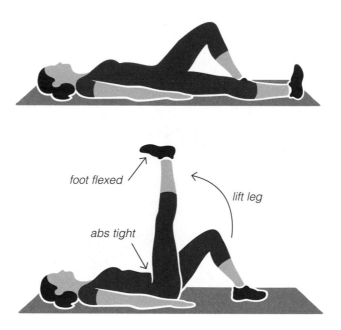

foot flexed

lift leg

abs tight

Bill Says: *If you lack mobility, you might start with a static stretch. Put a towel or strap over your foot, hold the ends with both hands, and use it to help raise your leg.*

Shoulder/Overhead Reach (Dry Backstroke)

Why Bother? This one is great for mid back and shoulder mobility. It stretches your pecs (the chest muscles in front that tend to pull you round-shouldered). Shoulder mobility is critical in life. Work on it or it goes away.

Step 1: Lie on your back with one or both legs bent. Reach over your head with one arm, touching the floor if you can. (Imagine a swimmer doing the backstroke.) Return the arm to your side. Keep your lower back quiet by tightening your abs.

Step 2: Extend the other arm, and continue to alternate between left and right, ten times each.

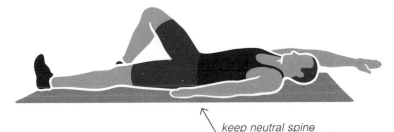

keep neutral spine

Bill Says: *Try these variations: 1) Do this with a foam-rubber roller vertically placed under your back; it lines up your spine nicely and works on your balance. (Google "foam rollers," or look around the gym.) 2) Try making "snow angels" in this same position.*

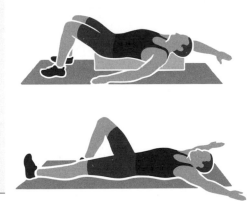

ON YOUR STOMACH

"I's" and "T's"

Why Bother? These enhance shoulder stability and mobility. They activate shoulder muscles and improve posture. In particular, they target the rotator cuff.

Step 1 ("I's"): Lie face-down on the floor or on a workout bench. Your head can be supported by a rolled-up towel or a small, calm dog (just kidding). With your arms at your sides, palms down, make the letter "I" with your body.

Step 2: Depress your shoulder blades back and down. With palms facing down, lift your arms until they are just above parallel with the floor. Contract your abs so lower back does not arch. Hold for three seconds. Slowly bring arms down until palms touch the floor. Repeat ten times.

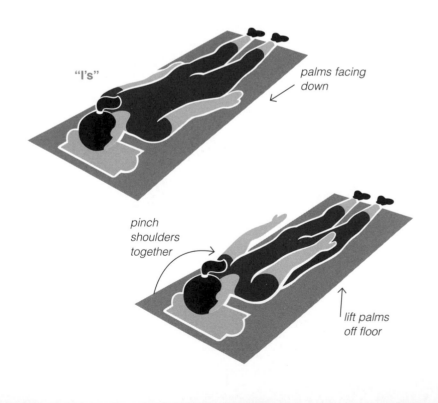

"I's"

palms facing down

pinch shoulders together

lift palms off floor

Step 3 ("T's"): Put your arms out to your sides, making a letter "T" with your body and head supported as described in Step 1. Depress your shoulder blades gently back and down; turn your arms so that your thumbs point upward. Tighten your abs, then lift your arms until they are just above parallel with the floor. Hold for three seconds. Slowly return your arms to the floor. Repeat ten to fifteen times.

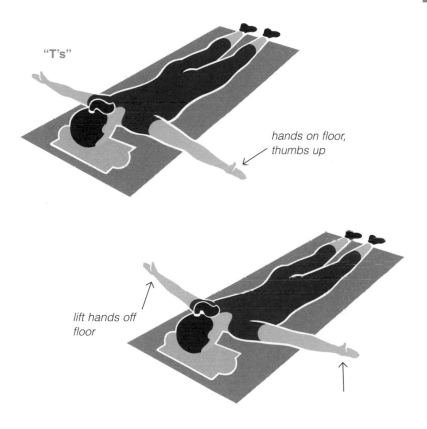

"T's"

hands on floor, thumbs up

lift hands off floor

Bill Says: *If you have shoulder issues,* do not skip this exercise.

ON YOUR SIDE
Side Leg Lift

Why Bother? This one activates your outer hip muscles to maintain alignment with single leg activities such as walking.

Step 1: Lie on your side with both legs fully extended, feet flexed (pull toes up). Look down to see if your body is in a straight line; do not bend from the hip. Squeeze the glutes and engage the abs. Lift your top leg about twelve inches off the floor. Hold five seconds. You should feel it right above your hip.

Step 2: Lower your leg and repeat the movement ten times on each side.

Too Easy? If you want more of a challenge, use a rubber band around your ankles.

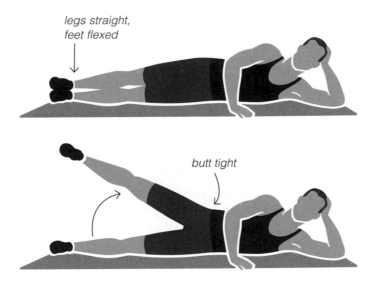

legs straight,
feet flexed

butt tight

Bill Says: *There's no need to try to raise the leg high.*

ON ALL FOURS

Cat and Camel

Why Bother? This one lubricates, warms, and loosens all the many joints in your back. If you have knee issues, use a foam pad or towel under your knees.

Step 1: Get on all fours, in a tabletop position. Hips over your knees and hands under shoulders. Slowly round the low and mid back by tilting the pelvis (camel). Hold for two or three seconds.

Step 2: Reverse into the opposite direction. Arch your back, stick out your tail and gently lift your neck and head (cat). Hold for two or three seconds. Repeat ten times.

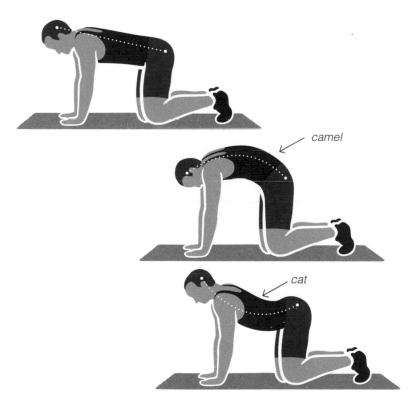

camel

cat

Hip Extension

Why Bother? Most of us are imbalanced, with tight hip flexors on the front of our hips and weak glutes on the backside. This exercise helps rebalance the length and activation of these muscles. If you have lost some hip mobility, do more of these.

Step 1: On all fours, extend the heel of one leg (with the knee flexed to 90 degrees) to the ceiling. Keep your lower back still by engaging your core muscles. Do ten reps at a slow to moderate speed. No jerky movements.

Step 2: Remember that your hip moves, but your back doesn't. Repeat with the other leg.

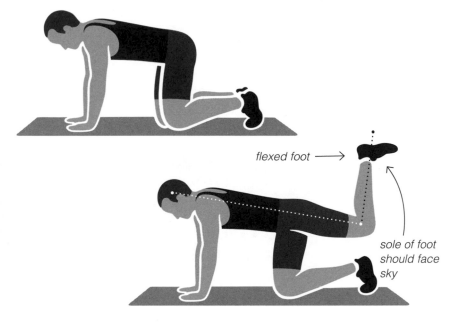

flexed foot ⟶

sole of foot should face sky

Bill Says: *If your hip is tight from years of sitting at a desk or from doing exercises that emphasize the flexed position, you need this one.*

Opposing Arm and Leg Reach

Why Bother? This addresses core stability, hip and shoulder mobility, and balance. A great exercise, and a little harder than it looks. Really reach for it, in both directions.

Step 1: In a tabletop position, tighten your abs to keep your low back quiet. Then reach way out with one arm and reach way back with the opposite leg. Hold for three to five seconds.

Activate all the muscles of the core, hip, and shoulder girdle.

Step 2: Return your hand and foot to the floor. Keep your hips level and your back still. This exercise is best done by alternating between your left and right sides. Do only four reps.

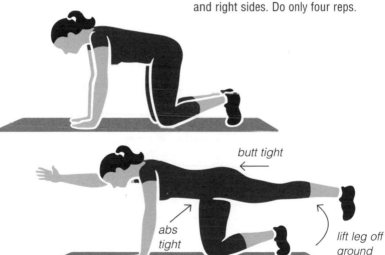

butt tight

abs tight

lift leg off ground

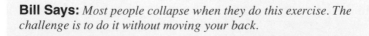

Bill Says: *Most people collapse when they do this exercise. The challenge is to do it without moving your back.*

Middle Back Mobility Turn

Why Bother? This stretch will loosen your mid back, an area where everyone tends to stiffen as they age. It is designed to offset the evil consequences of *slouching* your whole life.

Step 1: Start on all fours, then drop your butt down to your ankles. Put your left hand behind your head. Turn your upper body slowly to the right, looking over your right shoulder. Then turn your shoulder girdle to the left, opening up the body, as shown at right.

Step 2: With your right hand behind your head turn to the left. Do ten on each side. Try to increase range with each repetition.

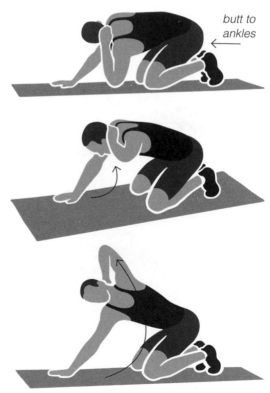

butt to ankles

Bill Says: *Mid back mobility is essential for both good shoulder mobility and to take loads off our low back. This is a must exercise.*

Hip Circles

Why Bother? Moving in three dimensions here is a great defensive move in the struggle to maintain the glass box.

Step 1: On all fours, lift one leg out to the side, then back, up, and down in a circular motion. Do ten clockwise on one side, then ten counterclockwise. Keep the low back still. As your mobility improves over time, increase the size of your circles.

Step 2: Repeat on the other side.

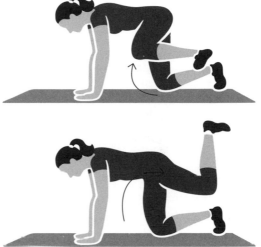

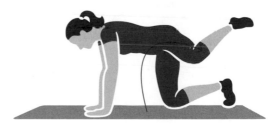

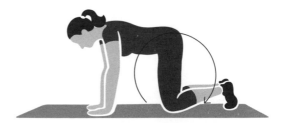

HALF-KNEELING

Half-Kneeling Stretch

Why Bother? This one does it all: hip and shoulder mobility, core stabilization, balance, and improved stability.

Step 1: Kneel down with one knee on the floor and the other leg bent and out in front. (You may want to put a towel or foam pad under the knee.) Set your posture: shoulders back and down, abs and glutes contracted. Shift your weight forward onto your front leg while lifting your arms overhead. Keep your spine in alignment. You should feel a stretch on the front of your rear leg (quad). Hold for three to five seconds.

Step 2: Bring arms back to your sides and shift your weight to your rear leg. Do ten reps on each side.

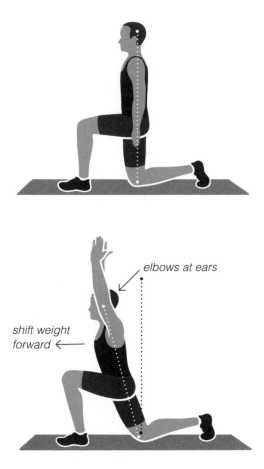

elbows at ears

shift weight forward ←

STANDING

Ankle Flex

Why Bother? This is a key exercise to prevent or reverse limited ankle mobility. Good ankle mobility is so important in climbing up or walking down stairs, doing squats and lunges—and so much else. And when it goes, it raises hell with everything else.

Step 1: Stand facing a wall. Bring one foot about six inches from the wall. Bend the knee slightly. Your back leg should be about a foot or two behind your front leg (the one being stretched). Put both hands against the wall. Try to drop most of your weight onto the flexed front foot. Keep your heel down and drive your knee over the front of that foot. Keep your feet facing straight ahead and do not let your heel come up or slide inward. Do ten reps.

Step 2: Switch sides and repeat. As you get better, place the front foot farther back from the wall.

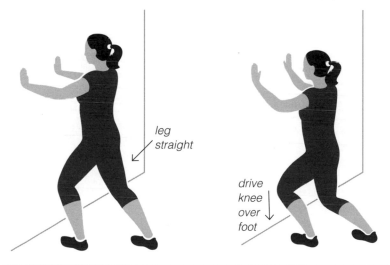

leg straight

drive knee over foot

Bill Says: *Don't be surprised if one ankle is more mobile than the other. You want to improve that asymmetry, because over time it can lead to a whole host of musculoskeletal problems.*

Balance on One Leg

Why Bother? One of the things we lose as we age, balance, can improve quickly and dramatically with practice. Better balance reduces the risk of falling.

Step 1: Stand tall; activate your quads, glutes, and abs. Move your shoulders back and down, and keep your chest lifted. Spread your arms out wide and lift one foot a few inches off the floor; try to maintain your balance for fifteen seconds. Repeat on the other foot.

Step 2: When you can hold for fifteen seconds, challenge yourself more. First, drop your hands to your sides. Next, try closing your eyes. For the ultimate balance challenge, try swinging the lifted leg back and forth and from side to side. Your balance will improve.

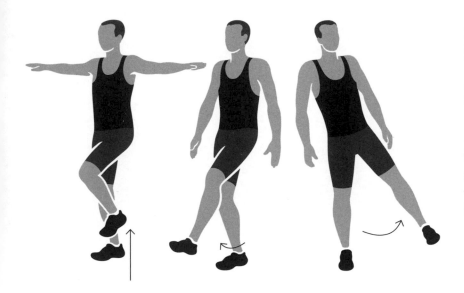

Bill Says: *You can improve your balance by doing exercises that require balance, such as squats and lunges.*

Squat and Reach

Why Bother? This is the time to get your body working as a unit and to groove some of the basic movements.

Step 1: Stand tall, with your feet facing forward and shoulder-width apart. Reach to the ceiling with your arms as high as they can go. Really reach.

Step 2: Bring your arms down and extend them out in front of you. Bend your hips and knees, and move into a squat by dropping your butt back and down. Go only as deep as you can while maintaining the alignment of your spine. Don't round over and don't let knees go forward of toes.

Step 3: Stand tall again; reach to the ceiling and squat again. Remember that your knees should track over your feet.

Bill Says: *When squatting, do not round your lower back, no matter what. Look straight ahead and keep your chest up.*

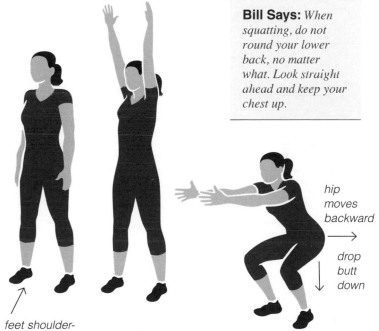

hip
moves
backward

drop
butt
down

feet shoulder-
width apart

Squat with Weight Shift

Why Bother? In the process of shifting your center of gravity you fire up your hip and knee muscles, enhance balance, and improve your hip mobility. Great for skiers, golfers, and all of us who simply need to expand our range of movement.

Step 1: Stand with your feet double shoulder-width apart. Squat down halfway, arms reaching forward. Then shift your weight over to either the left or the right leg, bending that knee and hip farther. Reach arms to the side and out over the foot that bears your weight. Keep your feet facing forward because you need to rotate around your hips.

Step 2: Shift your weight over to the other leg, now bending that knee and reaching forward with your arms. Then reach out to the side, with your arms over the foot onto which you've shifted your weight.

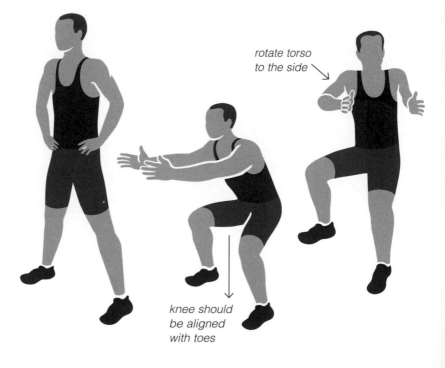

rotate torso to the side

knee should be aligned with toes

Fast Footwork

Why Bother? You may look a little like the monster in *Young Frankenstein* dancing to "Puttin' on the Ritz" but remember his joy, and keep dancing. Foot speed and coordination are key in the good life. Olympic athletes spend a huge amount of time on footwork; you should, too.

Step 1: Start with simple marching in place for ten seconds. Lift your knees high. Pump your arms. Start slow; get fast.

Step 2: Do this same high stepping for another ten seconds, at speed. Go for it. As you get more at home with this, add a little bounce to your step until you are jogging in place. Try skipping.

Step 3: When you really get into it (if you do), consider springing from side to side (see illustration on page 111). Someday, we hope, your feet are going to be flying.

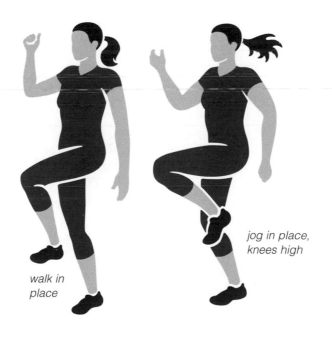

walk in place

jog in place, knees high

A Cold Day in Hell

I used to think, *It'll be a cold day in hell when I start doing warm-up exercises for pleasure.* That day finally arrived.

It took a while, but I finally drank the Kool-Aid on warming up, Bill's way. In the early days, these warm-ups seemed both too hard and too easy. And mildly annoying, for some reason. Mostly because they were "new," I suspect. Old boys and new tricks, man: It's an endless battle to make yourself open up to new stuff. I have come to revel in the "whole-body" feel of these warm-ups, the satisfying sense that I am pushing back on the walls of my own glass box.

When I first started, I looked like a dope doing lunges. My legs were strong, so how could that be? The answer, of course, is that although my major muscles were okay, the support muscles and my balance were less so. Doing lunges correctly—with a neutral spine and your chest up and looking straight ahead—is not so easy. I kept tumbling awkwardly to the left or the right. And I didn't like that. I wanted to go back to my machines, which I could do, because they're easier.

But Bill convinced me (slowly) that strength without balance did not amount to much. He persuaded me that usable strength meant whole-body strength. The kind you actually use when you ski or climb a hill. I needed more range of motion and better balance. The day I "got it" was my fifth time doing Bill's warm-up program, and the exercises started to feel natural and comfortable. And suddenly—and this is the miracle part—they didn't hurt as much. When I began, there were sharp twinges in my hips and shoulders, not major pain, but enough to tell me that I had not been using these joints. Then those twinges eased. Now there are none. I can reach way up and way down more easily. Even a bit gracefully, I think. And no pain. And not only in the gym. I have begun to notice, in my regular life, that I don't have as many twinges either. A miracle.

These warm-up exercises are primarily dynamic rather than static. That is, you move in and out of the stretch over several repetitions rather than holding it statically for too long. Think of the hip extensions, the straight leg raises, and so on—constant movement

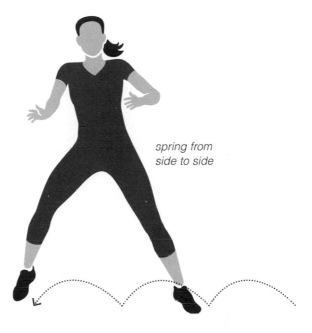

spring from side to side

Bill Says: *This exercise takes advantage of the remarkable springlike quality of muscles. They are rubber bands: You stretch them and they give you a pop of energy and propulsion. You do not get this as effectively on a treadmill or elliptical machine. Eventually, you will want to inject some side-to-side motion into these steps. Try laterally shuffling a few yards to the left and then to the right like a tennis player on the baseline. Great for all types of sports and life in general.*

to lengthen the tissue, repetition after repetition. They are great for joint mobility, coordination, muscle activation, and signaling. And they do not undermine muscle tone the way static stretches can.

Okay, you are officially and fully warmed up. Catch your breath. Turn back to the aerobic exercise section in Chapter Two or forward to the strength-training workout in Chapter Ten. You are so ready.

Strength Training: The Twenty-Five Sacred Exercises

Our goal here—Bill Fabrocini's goal, I should say—is to show you how to do the Twenty-Five Sacred Exercises that will be the foundation of all you need to know on the subject of strength training for the rest of your life. You may want to learn more eventually, but this will be the rock on which you build any regimen. Learn to do these twenty-five right, and you will know all the basic movements. Learn to do these right, and you will be able to walk into any gym in the country and know exactly what you're doing. Learn to do these right, and you will get into great shape and stay there. You can do these on your own perfectly well, and without much gear.

No Special Toys Required

There are four or five exercises where Bill suggests the use of gym machines. Use them if you've got them, but don't worry if you don't. All the exercises can be done with basic gear—very basic gear, like elastic bands and free weights. Elastic bands or tubes are wonderful gadgets and can be used instead of cables (wherever we mention cables). They come in different strengths (degrees of difficulty), coded by color. So if we say to increase weight on a machine, just increase resistance with a more difficult elastic tubing. You can buy three of them and have a decent gym. This is not about money; it's about technique. Having said that, we think a gym membership (or membership at the local YMCA or community gym) is always a great idea, if there's a decent one nearby. (See "Join a Gym," page 34.)

We illustrate each exercise using what we think of as the best equipment for it. But a moment's thought will make it possible to do almost all of them with some combination of elastic bands and free weights.

Repetition and Range of Motion

Drill yourself a little on the exercises; repetition is of the essence. But once you get them grooved—once they move into your muscle memory—you will have them forever and they will seem automatic. And they will do all the amazing things that we promise will come to you with serious strength training. You're going to go through the exercises a number of times before you get them; it's taken me awhile. But I did get them and you will, too. And hard to believe now, but it gets to be *almost* fun, after a while.

Bill has a couple of rules of general application:

RULE 1: Do these exercises for several repetitions—ten to twelve typically—but always stop at "failure." For Bill "failure" has a special meaning. It means do them until you *fail to do them right*. Then stop. If you can't maintain a neutral spine on a squat—if your knee starts to buckle on a lunge—if your head pops forward or your shoulders hunch on a pull-down—stop! That's the new failure. Go on to the next exercise. Or do an easier version of that one. But don't do them wrong; that's less than useless. You can get hurt.

In traditional strength training, "going to failure" meant lifting heavier and heavier loads until you just couldn't do another rep because your muscles hurt too much. That still makes sense, but Bill wants you to see failure in a different light. Here's Bill on the subject: "I cannot tell you how many clients I've had who got in trouble by ignoring good form and going to failure, the old-fashioned way, but with their bodies in poor alignment. It was as if they were deliberately hurting themselves. I have seen serious weight lifters with severe degenerative backs, worn-down knees, and dreadful hip problems all from doing strength training with bad alignment. *Never overload dysfunction.* In other words, if you can't perform these exercises correctly, don't add more weight or try to do them with speed. It is a painfully common mistake. Our joints and backs are engineering miracles. But they will not stand up to decades of off-center pressures that come with bad posture and faulty movement. Bad strength training is much, much worse than none at all."

RULE 2: Use full range of motion (or try to) on every exercise. You may not be able to do this on a lot of these exercises at first. Or maybe ever. But trying to do so keeps the glass box from shrinking. Reach all the way up, all the way down; squat until your thighs are parallel to the ground. Those are the moves that are going to preserve range of motion in your joints. Full range of motion—or the closest you can get to it—is always the goal. And think PSM (Posture, Stability, Movement) whenever you work out.

Why should you care about full range of motion for, say, your quads?

The answer to that may become painfully obvious. Think falling down. When you fall down, you get full range of motion in

---

♆ *THE DOCTOR IS IN:* On Falling

You're much more likely to fall as you get older unless you stay in great shape. Falls have been carefully studied, and it turns out that you do not stumble much more often as you age, and you catch your toe about as often as you did at twenty. But instead of easily recovering your balance, you're more likely to hit the pavement. Why? Well, the neurotransmitters that coordinate balance deteriorate with age. After all, simple walking is really a series of near falls followed by a million tiny adjustments and recovery. When you age, the wiring that manages all that falls apart, and you no longer catch yourself. It takes a split second longer before your brain realizes you're falling, and in that split second, momentum and gravity turn against you. The other point is that it takes strength to recover from a stumble. Your toe stops on the pavement, but your body keeps going, building up speed and momentum in a Newtonian drive toward earth. Your legs have to be strong enough to stop your momentum, or down you go. And if you've happened to let your bones decay, and have osteoporosis, down you stay.

Lifting weights fixes up the wiring and helps cure the problem. Not a hundred percent, but near. If you do take a fall, having strong reflexes and powerful muscles changes it from a head-on collision to a softer impact. You will fall less if you're strong, and you will fall better, dramatically lowering your odds of serious injury.

your quads in a heartbeat. You go all the way down to a right angle and beyond. And if you don't have strength in your legs in that range, you will keep on going down until you crash in a heap. Maybe a painful heap because you did not have good range of motion.

Range of motion involves muscle strength, but more important is range of motion in your joints. Eighty percent of people over fifty have lost significant mobility (range of motion) in their hips or their ankles. Eighty percent have lost mobility in their back. A vast number have lost mobility in their shoulder joints. Good range of motion matters for all kinds of things. If you lose mobility in your shoulder, you will not be able to reach all the way up on the shelf to get the vodka bottle down. (Tip: Do *not* solve this problem by lowering the vodka bottle—that's cheating.) If you lose mobility in your ankles (a painfully common thing), you simply will not be able to walk right. And your hips will start to get funny. And that in turn will cause your back to go. It's not all a matter of being able to ski the bumps. It's a matter of getting the cereal off the shelf, walking naturally. Range of motion counts. Joint mobility counts tremendously. The glass box counts.

Falls aside, strength training lowers your chance of injury with all forms of exercise—in large part by speeding up your reflexes, but also by strengthening your tendons, ligaments, and joints. Tendons and ligaments are living tissue, but they atrophy as you get older. Pulling hard on a tendon strengthens the nerve connections and makes the tendon grow a bit farther into the bone, strengthening the attachment and rendering it more resistant to injury. Good for your joints! Good for you.

All of which should happen once you become proficient in our first exercise, squats. Doing squats looks easy and obvious. It is neither. It is hugely important to do them correctly (especially with a neutral spine and with good alignment) and eventually to achieve a "full range of motion." Squats, that is, dropping down so your thighs are parallel to the floor, are truly basic. Learn to do them right, and do a lot of them—with or without weights—for the rest of your life. It will keep you moving with strength and a touch of grace, forever.

STARTING OUT WITH WEIGHTS: In the first few weeks or months, start with weights that are "too light" so you can be sure to do the exercises correctly. In other words, do less weight than you can handle and more repetitions—maybe twenty instead of ten to twelve. Give your joints time to get into the game and your body time to focus on technique and alignment. Do not over-muscle your joints. Add more weight slowly, as you get better at the exercises. Have someone give you feedback about your posture or check your own alignment in the gym mirror. Develop that all-important "muscle memory."

General Rules for All Exercises

Eventually your goal is to do ten to twelve reps per set, and two or three sets of reps. Except where it says otherwise, do them slowly, on both sides or in both directions. As you get more technically proficient with these exercises, that is, you're able to do them with less conscious effort, add weight. Eventually you have to go heavier and do fewer repetitions. Until you can do only, say, eight reps on the third set. This is strength training, in the end. This is the war on sarcopenia. This is building and maintaining muscle. And you do not do that without resistance, and eventually, some muscle pain. Learn to do these correctly, then gradually push yourself to add more weight.

It is not the plan to have you do all twenty-five substantive exercises every strength-training day; it would take too long. You should always do the Warm-ups first. (Bill says, don't cut corners here.) Then do *a selection of the twenty-five strength exercises.* You may pick and choose within the exercises here, as long as you do some from each category. For example, do a couple of lower body and a couple of upper body, one rotation, and at least one combination exercise. A forty-five-minute (total) strength day is plenty. Bill suggests that you stay with the same set of exercises for two to three weeks, until you master it and then change it up. Exercises from different categories are designed to work together.

Your muscles need a day or two to recover, so spread out your strength-training sessions. (See a typical Weekly Plan, page 157.)

Once you learn to do these correctly and get into decent shape, you may want to do some of them (especially the advanced compound exercises) with more speed. Doing those exercises—which recruit a large number of muscles—at speed is a tremendous aerobic workout as well. Engaging a whole bunch of muscles means a whole bunch of mitochondria—a huge burn.

A Word About Intensity and Difficulty

We focus a lot on technique in this chapter and on showing you how to get the movements right. There is less emphasis on increasing the intensity. As I've said earlier, the way you get stronger and more fit is by stressing your muscles. You do that by making the exercises progressively harder over time. So once you've mastered technique, you will want to turn your attention to gradually increasing the degree of difficulty. That is how you stress your muscles enough to turn decay into growth, or how to cause enough C-6 to trigger C-10.

How do you do it? You add resistance, increase weight. You increase challenges to balance. Or you increase speed. For example, Bill is very detailed about how to do squats and lunges correctly. Eventually, you are going to want to make them harder by using weights. You can hold a dumbbell in each hand or a weight under your chin as you do them. Or do squats on uneven surfaces (a BOSU Trainer, for example) to make them harder because you constantly need to adjust your balance. (You will not want to add speed to those.)

Toward the end, Bill shows you some complex rotational exercises, using either a medicine ball (great device), machines (the cable machine in the gym is a "good" machine), or the TRX Rip Trainer. It takes awhile to learn to use the Rip Trainer correctly. But one of the joys of this device is that you can use it hard and fast to do basic movements—and give yourself a great strength and aerobic workout at the same time. All the while you're expanding your glass box. Do it slowly till you get the technique just right. Then (when you're in shape) do it as hard as you can for, say, thirty seconds. Killer!

You may not want to, but eventually you should crank it up, focus on stressing the body more and more. This has to get hard in order to work. Like life, I suppose. Annoying.

Don't Try to Do All of These from the Get-Go

This is a pretty serious strength-training regimen, and it is going to take awhile to get comfortable with it. Hell, it's going to take awhile to be able to do it at all. **One suggestion is just to focus on the relatively easy ones first (marked with an asterisk*).** Then work your way into the others. Stay with the starred exercises for a week or two—whatever suits you. Feel your way. Even experienced trainers find some of these hard at first. Don't make yourself crazy. Last tip: Read these strength chapters over again, from time to time. I do, and I wrote 'em. Different points will resonate as you get into it.

Eventually, you'll want to do a thorough, balanced strength workout, one that covers your lower body, your core (back and abs), and your upper body.

Two things that I learned the hard way and that may reassure you. One: These exercises are easier than they look when you read about them. Two: Some of these are harder than they look. For heaven's sake, don't feel compelled to do all of them right away. If some defeat you at first, fine! Skip them and go on to the others. Twenty-five exercises like these turn out to be quite a few. Do not force yourself to learn them all at once. Pick your way through; get into it gradually. Supplement the new workouts with the old (machine) stuff, if you like. You are not preparing for an exam next week; you're preparing for life. Take your time. Learn to do the easier ones (with asterisks) correctly. Go on to the rest over time.

Download a nine-page illustrated cheat sheet for the Twenty Five Sacred Exercises, and order the Strength-Training DVD at youngernextyear.com.

NUMBER 1

Squat*

Why Bother? Superb exercise for strengthening your core and the big muscles of your legs. This is one of the basic movements in life.

Step 1: With your core tightened and your back straight, drop your butt back and down until it almost touches the chair behind you. Hinge from the hips. Keep a nice straight spine, and make sure your knees are tracking over your feet.

Step 2: Return to standing.

Do It Right. When your spine starts to round or your knees wobble or your head pops forward, stop.

Too Difficult? Don't go all the way down.

Too Easy? Hold a dumbbell in each hand at your side.

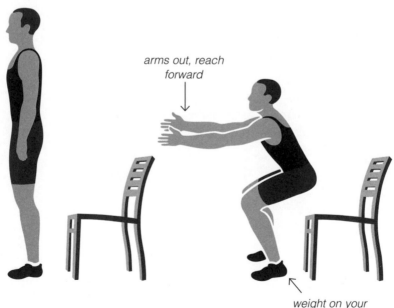

arms out, reach forward

weight on your heels

STRENGTH TRAINING

NUMBER 2

Split Squat*

Why Bother? This version adds a touch of asymmetry and so demands more balance. Bill thinks it is *the* great strength-training move. It is great for hip stability, loss of which leads to many ills. Ditto, of course, for balance.

Step 1: Stand with one foot about eighteen inches ahead of the other, with your weight more or less evenly balanced. With the front leg, flex the hips and knees; lower your butt until your front thigh is parallel to the floor. Flex your back leg toward the floor.

Step 2: Ascent: Drive upward with the emphasis on your front leg, pushing through the heel. Keep an even tempo, with a count of down 1, 2, 3 and up 1, 2, 3.

Do It Right. When your spine starts to round or your knee dives into the midline, stop. You have done it to failure.

Too Easy? Put your hands behind your head. This helps you maintain good posture by keeping your back upright. Eventually, you may want to add weights in each hand.

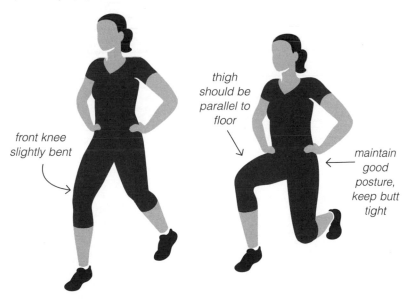

front knee slightly bent

thigh should be parallel to floor

maintain good posture, keep butt tight

NUMBER 3

Single-Leg Squat

Equipment Needed: None, unless you are a mere human, in which case you may need something to hang on to. The wall, the TRX Suspension Strap, whatever. Bill admits that "top athletes struggle with this one." Few will be able to do an unaided, single-leg squat for quite a while, if ever. But that's okay.

Why Bother? It leads to amazing hip stability and ferrets out and corrects imbalance. Being out of balance is serious, and compensating for it makes it worse. Asymmetrical exercises—especially extreme ones like this—correct weakness. No way to compensate for a bum hip when you're standing on one leg. Learn to do some version of these. They are hard but wonderful for you.

Step 1: Standing in front of a bench or chair, lift one foot slightly off the floor. Descend by bending your knee and hip so that your butt moves back and descends as close as it can to the bench or chair. Note: Very few will be able to do more than a shallow squat. But the goal is the same.

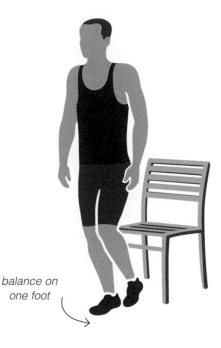

balance on one foot

Step 2: Ascend as before. Go slowly and with control.

Do It Right. Remember to maintain a neutral spine and alignment and don't let your knee buckle inward toward the midline. Go only as far as you can correctly.

Too Difficult? Tap your raised foot on the floor, as needed. You can also do these near a wall with your hip descending and moving backward until it touches the wall, for support.

Too Easy? If you think this is too easy, you have stumbled into the wrong book. But you can crank it up with weights.

try to get your butt as close to the chair as you can without sitting on it

Bill Says: *There is nothing like asymmetrical movement to improve hip stability, balance, coordination, and strength of the stressed leg and of the core.*

STRENGTH TRAINING

NUMBER 4

The Lunge*

Equipment Needed: None. (You may want to use the TRX Suspension Strap for balance in the early stages, or maybe a pair of ski poles.)

Why Bother? I personally think this is the single best exercise in the book. Great for hip stability, leg and core strength, and balance.

Step 1: Stand with your feet in a fairly narrow stance, keeping a neutral spine and good alignment. On the descent, step forward approximately two feet (less if you are short) and lower your body as in a squat. Have your knee track directly over your foot. Goal: To bring your front thigh parallel to the floor. It may take a while. Do the best you can.

Step 2: On the ascent, drive up with your hips and knees, pushing through the heel. Maintain a neutral spine and upright (aligned) posture throughout. You can also do walking lunges— lunge all around the gym. Or lunge in place.

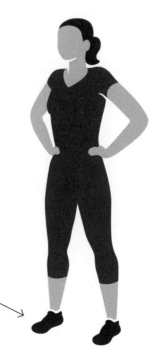

narrow stance

Do It Right. It is of the essence in this exercise to maintain a neutral spine and good alignment. And to quit when you cannot or if your knees start to wobble or buckle.

Too Difficult? Don't drop down as deep. Use the devices (mentioned in headnote) to steady you.

Too Easy? As you get better, move the center of gravity up by putting your hands behind your head. Add weights—either dumbbells in each hand or a single weight (dumbbell or medicine ball) in both hands, held just under the chin. Or try the lunge by stepping backward.

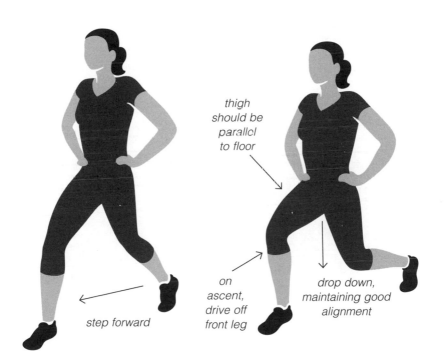

thigh should be parallel to floor

on ascent, drive off front leg

step forward

drop down, maintaining good alignment

STRENGTH TRAINING

NUMBER 5

Lateral Lunge*

Equipment Needed: Same as the lunge.

Why Bother? This one has added benefits in terms of hip stability and unilateral leg strength, which you need all the time. Side-to-side movement is the point here.

Step 1: Start with your feet in a fairly narrow stance. Step to one side, as far as you comfortably can (a couple of feet is fine), shifting your body weight to the supporting leg. (Keep your feet facing forward.) Lower your body as in a squat while extending the arms forward. Your hips will shift back during the descent.

Step 2: Push up, primarily with the laterally placed leg, and return to a narrow stance.

Too Difficult? Hang on to something in the early stages. Do not drop as deep.

Too Easy? Hold a dumbbell in both hands under your chin or between your legs.

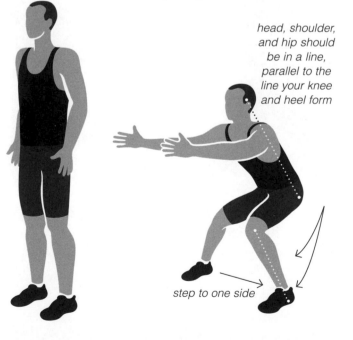

head, shoulder, and hip should be in a line, parallel to the line your knee and heel form

step to one side

NUMBER 6

Pull Down* (with Machine)

Why Bother? Helps to strengthen your shoulder girdle muscles and enhances back stabilization.

Step 1: Set weights at a light level. Sit down and seize the bar, with your palms facing away and hands shoulder-width apart (arms fully extended overhead). Depress your shoulder blades and slowly pull the bar down to your chest. (Variations: Try a wider or narrower grip or have palms facing inward.)

Step 2: Slowly return the bar, until your arms are stretched fully overhead, using controlled movement all the way. This is a range-of-motion improvement exercise. Feel your way toward a level where doing ten to twelve reps is demanding.

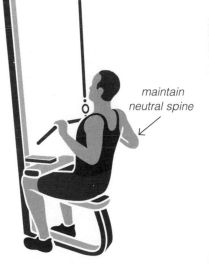

don't
drop
head
forward

maintain
neutral spine

STRENGTH TRAINING

NUMBER 7

One-Armed Dumbbell Row*

Equipment Needed: A gym bench, but any chair or bench will do, plus dumbbells suitable for you.

Why Bother? This one improves your one-arm pulling strength, enhances the strength of your shoulder girdle, improves your core stabilization, and teaches you to control rotational strength of your body.

Step 1: Kneel with one knee on a bench and the other foot on the floor. Support yourself with your arm on the bench. Pick up dumbbell.

Step 2: With extended arm grasping the dumbbell, pull shoulder girdle back, then drive elbow toward the ceiling. Pull dumbbell upward to just above the hip.

Do It Right. Maintain a neutral spine throughout the movement. Don't hunch.

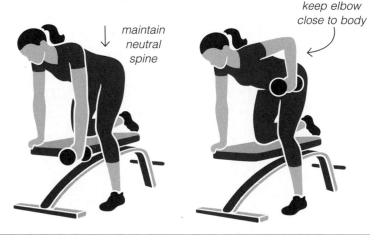

↓ maintain neutral spine

keep elbow close to body

Bill Says: *To create a balanced body, single-arm exercises like this one help.*

NUMBER 8

One-Armed Cable Row*

Why Bother? Does the same for upper-body strength as the previous exercise but uses more of the whole body.

Equipment Needed: The Cable Machine is one of the best machines in the gym because of the angle of the pull and its ability to increase or decrease weights easily. And it allows full range of motion.

Cross-Linkage. The body is naturally "cross-linked" to facilitate movement across the body, lower right to upper left and vice versa.

Step 1: Set a cable machine with the grip close to the floor. Start with a light weight and feel your way. With one leg forward in a split squat (see Number 2), grasp the handle with the opposite hand; if your left foot is forward, use your right hand. Depress shoulder girdle and pull the handle to your side in a single-arm row. Pull until hand is just above right hip.

Step 2: Slowly return to starting position. Use controlled movement.

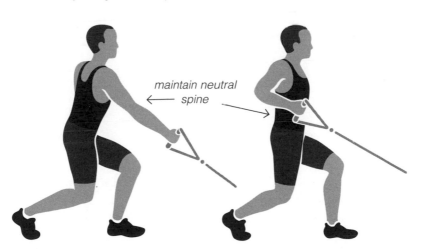

maintain neutral
← spine →

NUMBER 9

Chest Press (Bench)*

Equipment Needed: A padded gym bench, but any bench will do.

Why Bother? There comes a time in life when you have to push back! This helps. It also enhances your shoulder girdle and core.

Step 1: This is, in effect, a push-up off a bench. Lean over the bench, arms fully extended and your body straight. Bend elbows and slowly lower yourself until your upper body almost touches the bench. Alignment is most important here. Don't let shoulders collapse or belly sag.

Step 2: Push up until your arms are straight again.

Do It Right. Be particularly careful to maintain a neutral spine while doing chest presses. Do these right or don't do them at all.

Too Difficult? Try doing the chest press against a door or wall. The nearer you are to the wall, the shallower the push-up and the easier it is to stay in alignment.

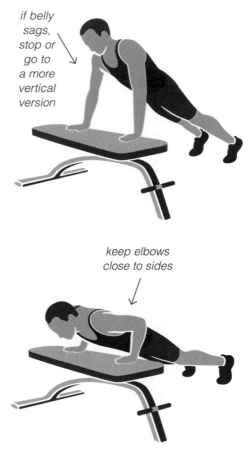

if belly sags, stop or go to a more vertical version

keep elbows close to sides

STRENGTH TRAINING

NUMBER 10

Single-Arm Dumbbell Press*

Equipment Needed: A padded bench (you can probably cobble one up at home). And a dumbbell.

Why Bother? This one enhances your "push strength" and core strength and helps stabilize your shoulder girdle. Also good for your "lats," the big lateral muscles that run down your back in a "V." The unbalanced feature does the usual, wonderful things.

Step 1: Lie on your back on a padded bench, feet flat and spread wide on the floor. Keep some arch in your back. (You may need a box or other lift under your feet so your lower back does not overarch.) Hold a dumbbell in one hand, slightly away from your body, at shoulder height.

Step 2: Engage abs and depress shoulder girdle. Push or drive the dumbbell upward, straight over the shoulder, toward the ceiling. Use an even tempo and the same count raising and lowering the weight. Don't snap your elbow into extension.

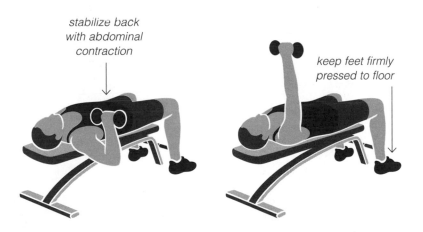

stabilize back with abdominal contraction

keep feet firmly pressed to floor

NUMBER 11

Single-Arm Cable Press*

Equipment Needed: Cable press machine or elastic tube.

Why Bother? This one has a bit more of the cross-linkage than the dumbbell press. It is great for shoulder, hip, and core stabilization, and trains rotational movement.

Step 1: Load the machine appropriately (start light, as always). Anchor the cable at a height midway between your waist and shoulders. Stand in a split-squat position (see Number 2), facing away from the machine.

Step 2: The movement is like throwing a punch. If the right leg is forward, take the cable in your left hand (back) at shoulder height. Punch forward with the left arm in a horizontal path and shift your weight onto the front foot. Return to starting position by bending your elbow and bringing your hand back to shoulder height. Do it slowly and with control.

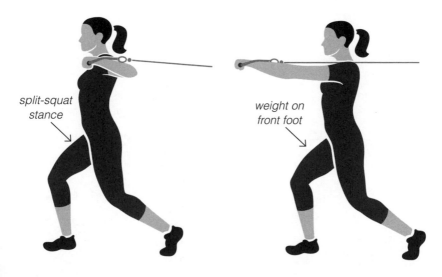

split-squat stance

weight on front foot

NUMBER 12

Split-Squat Overhead Press

Equipment Needed: Dumbbell or other weight.

Why Bother? It's great for the core. Skip this if you have shoulder issues.

Step 1: Assume the descent position of a split squat (see Number 2), with your knee bent, holding a dumbbell at shoulder height. If your right leg is forward, the dumbbell should be in your left hand.

Step 2: Ascend in the split-squat position while thrusting the dumbbell straight up and overhead. (A little upward thrust from the legs to create momentum is fine, but don't straighten the legs.)

Step 3: Return the dumbbell to your shoulder as you drop back down. Switch to the other side.

Do It Right. Like all asymmetrical exercises, this one is designed to throw you off balance. Don't let it.

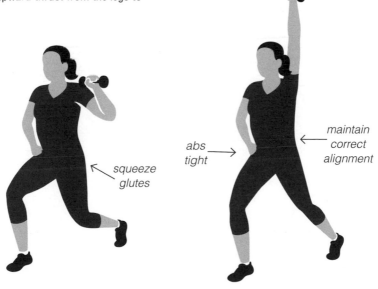

squeeze
glutes

abs
tight

maintain
correct
alignment

NUMBER 13

Rotation/Chop with Medicine Ball

Why Bother? One of my favorites. It's hard but a great exercise to stretch the glass box. Use a light medicine ball.

Step 1: Stand with your feet shoulder-width apart. Hold the medicine ball out in front of your body, arms slightly bent. Engage your abs. Begin squat position, moving down and to the right, bringing the ball around to the right. Squat and lower the ball as close as you can to the floor, without losing the neutral spine. Keep shoulders back. You may not be able to get much past your knees at first. Your body should move as a unit, facing the ball as you swing it to your right or left. *Rotate your hips, not your lower back. Your belly button should follow the ball!*

Step 2: Slowly swing the ball up to your waist and, without pausing, straight around to the left and over your shoulder, as high as you can reach. The ball follows a diagonal path, moving from outside your right foot to over your left shoulder, or vice versa. Remember: Rotate your hips, not your lower back, the same way you did on the way down. Return to starting position.

Do It Right. You can get hurt if you do this wrong. So do it right or do not do it at all. Rotate your hips, not your lower back. This is one of the fundamental lessons of this book. And maintain a neutral spine throughout.

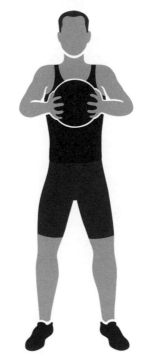

Too Difficult? Use less or no weight. Do not go as deep. Most of you will not be able to put the ball all the way down to the floor without losing the neutral spine. Don't!

Too Easy? Add weight, go deeper (touch the ball to the floor) but only if you can do it with a neutral spine.

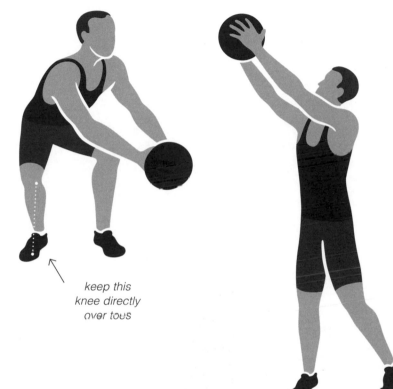

keep this knee directly over toes

Bill Says: *Feel your way with this one for a long time, focusing heavily on rotating your hips, following the ball (or your hands) with your belly button. Learn to move instinctively in this manner, and you will have done yourself a profound favor for life.*

NUMBER 14

Rotation/Chop with Cable Machine

Equipment Needed: Cable machine or elastic tube.

Why Bother? A variation of the medicine ball chop, but the resistance on the cable machine is applied at an angle directly through the rotational arc of movement.

Step 1: Set the cable machine with light weight; attach the pulley at the base near the floor. Stand sideways to the machine with handle in both hands, your whole body turned toward the machine. Drop into a squat, turning toward the anchor point as deeply as you can with a neutral spine.

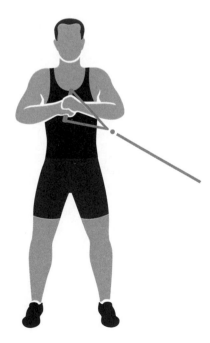

Step 2: Raise the handle up to your waist, and, in a single continuous movement, raise it up to your left and over your opposite shoulder, as high as you can reach. Maintain a neutral spine. Have belly button follow your hands, as in Number 13.

Too Difficult? Use less (or no) weight. Do not go down as deep.

Too Easy? Increase weight.

Bill Says: *It takes a while to get used to this movement. Don't worry about weight until you really have it down. And never go deeper down than you can go with a truly neutral spine or you can get hurt.*

STRENGTH TRAINING

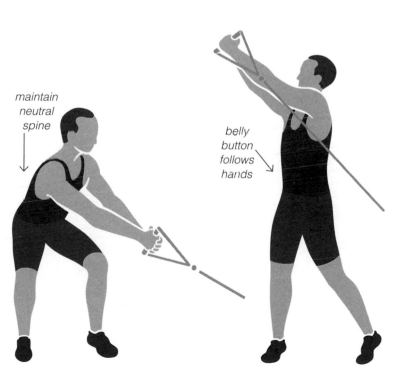

maintain neutral spine

belly button follows hands

NUMBER 15

Squat Single-Arm Overhead Press

Equipment Needed: Dumbbells. Start with what feels like too little weight. It will get heavy fast. Then adjust over time.

Why Bother? This one is all about the critical transfer of force—from the legs to the arms, from the lower to the upper body. It seems easy and obvious; it is what you were built for. But it helps develop the core (in rotation) and your unilateral (one-armed) coordination.

Step 1: Start with your feet shoulder-width (or slightly farther) apart, holding dumbbells (one in each hand) at shoulder level, palms facing forward. Descend into a squat position while maintaining a neutral spine; keep your knees in close alignment with your toes.

Step 2: Once you reach the low point of your squat, forcefully ascend

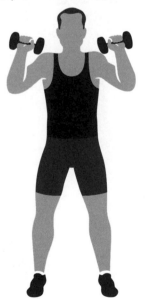

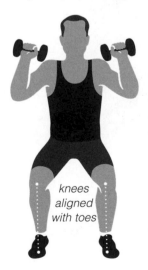

knees aligned with toes

back upward. As momentum builds, drive one arm (holding the dumbbell) directly up toward the ceiling. Finish by returning your arm and dumbbell to shoulder level.

Step 3: Repeat squat sequence, but this time, on the ascent, drive the opposite arm toward the ceiling. Finish by returning your arm to shoulder level in a standing position.

Too Difficult/Easy? Adjust weights.

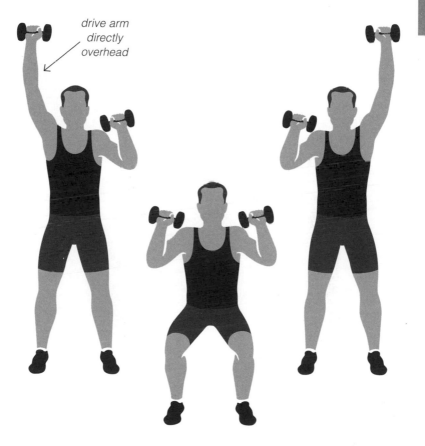

drive arm directly overhead

NUMBER 16

Back Step Lunge Row

Equipment Needed: Cable machine or elastic tube.

Why Bother? This is real whole-body stuff. It combines the split squat with a row and finishes with a backward lunge. Once you get the coordination down, you'll enjoy it.

Step 1: Set cable with anchor near floor, using a modest weight. Stand in a split squat (see Number 2) facing machine. Place your left foot forward and take the cable handle in your right hand, extended toward the machine.

Step 2: Begin by stepping forward with your back foot (in this case, the right). Do the step by driving upward with the front (or left) leg. Simultaneously, as you straighten your body to standing, pull your right arm toward your side, just above the hip. Finish in a narrow stance, with your right arm in a "row" position, shoulders back and elbow bent.

Step 3: Return to the start position by reaching forward with the right arm as you lunge back with your right foot, resuming the original split-squat position. Repeat on other side.

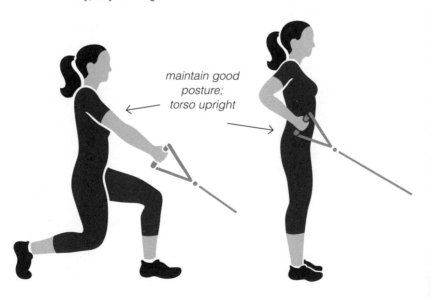

maintain good posture; torso upright

NUMBER 17

Squat, Arm Curl

Equipment Needed: Dumbbells. Again, start light so you can do them perfectly before going up in weight.

Why Bother? Here Bill has combined the "biceps curl" with a squat to get us away from the temptation to do this the old-fashioned way: by muscle isolation.

Step 1: Stand with your feet shoulder-width apart, holding a pair of dumbbells down at your sides. Descend into a squat with your arms extended, dumbbells in hands, moving toward the floor. Palms can be facing forward or inward, whichever is more comfortable.

Step 2: Rise out of the squat position, as you bend your arms so

the dumbbells move toward your shoulders. (Your wrists will flip 90 degrees so dumbbells face forward as you lift.) It is okay to use some momentum to swing the weights a bit on this one. But do not let your body buckle from side to side or get out of neutral alignment.

Step 3: Slowly return the weights to your sides.

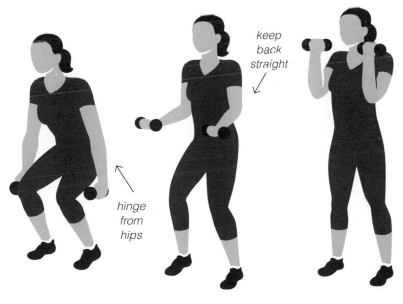

keep
back
straight

hinge
from
hips

STRENGTH TRAINING

NUMBER 18

Bend, Pull, Overhead Press

Equipment Needed: Dumbbells.

Why Bother? This is a basic lift. We pick stuff up off the floor and raise it to a counter or waist height. Or raise it to an upper shelf, over our heads. Do it right to prevent back pain.

Step 1: With legs at least shoulder-width apart, bend over and grab two dumbbells off the floor. Remember to hinge from your hips, with a neutral spine. The movement of bending over is less of a squat and more of a bend from the hips. Your knees can bend slightly, but the object is to keep them straighter. If you have very tight hamstrings, you may not be able to reach the floor without rounding your back. If this is the case, place the dumbbells on a box or other "lift" so you do not have to bend over as far.

Step 2: Engage your glutes and maybe stick your butt out to maintain a straight back. Straighten back up

hinge from hips

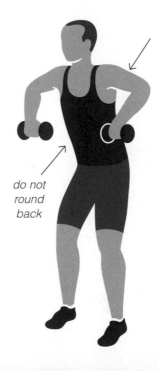

do not round back

while lifting the dumbbells off the floor. (Be careful not to round your lower back.) Simultaneously pull the dumbbells upward to shoulder height. Without pausing—and using the momentum already created—push the dumbbells directly over your head.

Step 3: Return the dumbbells to shoulder height, then bend over and reach down with your arms until the dumbbells touch the floor (or the lift) again. Repeat the entire sequence.

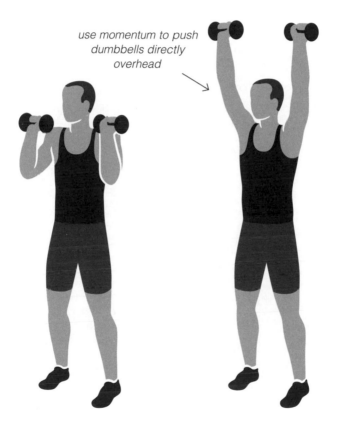

use momentum to push dumbbells directly overhead

Bill Says: *This reads harder than it is. Look at the pictures and try it a few times. Not bad.*

STRENGTH TRAINING

> **Specialized Exercises:** The next few exercises focus on specific areas of the body that folks often have issues with—such as shoulders and hips.

NUMBER 19

"I's" and "T's" with Dumbbells*

Equipment Needed: Light dumbbells, a padded bench to lie on.

Why Bother? These are great for your shoulder girdle, mid- and low-back stabilization, and strengthening your rotator cuff. Similar to the warm-up on pages 96 to 97, but much harder.

"I's"

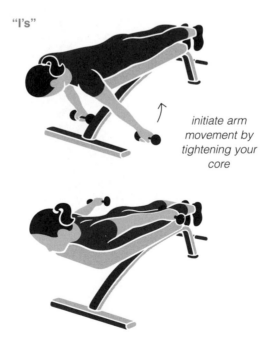

↑ *initiate arm movement by tightening your core*

Step 1: Lie on your stomach on a padded bench, keeping your head and chest just slightly off the bench. Hold dumbbells in both hands. For the "I's," lie with your arms at your sides and palms down. For the "T's," lie with your thumbs pointing up and your arms out to the sides.

Step 2: Gently lift your chest slightly off the bench, extending from the mid back, shoulders depressed (not hunched). Do not arch from the low back. Initiate the arm movement by tightening your core. Lift both arms (from the floor) to just higher than parallel with your body. Hold for three seconds. Slowly bring your arms back to the floor. Do ten I's and ten T's.

"T's"

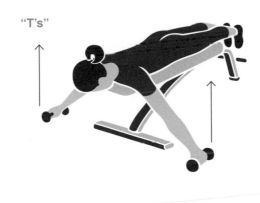

pinch shoulders
together

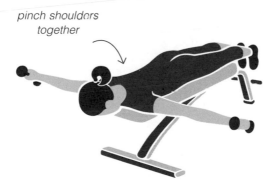

NUMBER 20

Rotator Cuff External Rotation with Dumbbell*

Equipment Needed: Foam pad, dumbbells—start very light.

Why Bother? This one is a beauty to build rotator cuff strength and enhance shoulder girdle stability.

Step 1: Lie on your right side with your hands as shown: left elbow at a 90-degree angle, forearm across your body. Grasp the weight. Keeping your elbow close to your side, slowly rotate your elbow 180 degrees so the dumbbell points up toward the ceiling. You will feel some muscle burn right behind your upper shoulder.

Step 2: Lower weight to starting position, slowly, over a count of four or five. This is very important to build strength. Repeat on the other side, with right arm.

Too Easy? In time, try to add resistance and lower the number of reps until you are able to do only, say, eight reps.

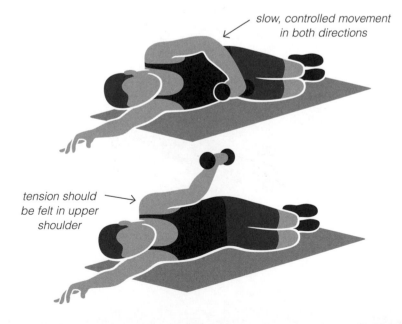

slow, controlled movement in both directions

tension should be felt in upper shoulder

NUMBER 21

Hip Extension Lift*

Equipment Needed: Foam pad, chair, or Swiss ball to rest your heels on. Be cautious with this exercise if you have knee problems.

Why Bother? Most of us, after forty or fifty, lose hip extension strength because we spend so much time in a "flexed" position, sitting at a desk. This exercise is a must for those with atrophied glutes (a nice way of saying "sagging butt").

Step 1: Lie on your back with your knees at a 90-degree angle, heels on a chair. Contract your abs and glutes. Drive your heels down on the chair—keeping feet flexed—and lift butt off the floor. Hold for three seconds. Slowly lower your body back down.

Too Difficult? Use a lower chair/bench or don't lift your butt as high.

Too Easy? Hold for five seconds. Use TRX Suspension Trainer stirrups (to add a balance component).

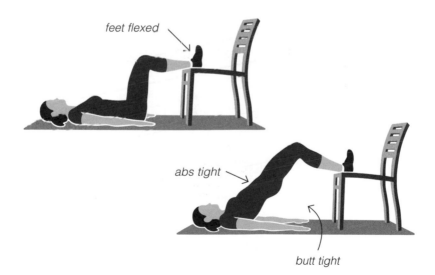

feet flexed

abs tight

butt tight

NUMBER 22

Plank*

Equipment Needed: Foam pad.

Why Bother? This one enhances hip, shoulder, and core stabilization, especially the core.

Step 1: Lie on your stomach, up on your elbows. Contract your glutes and abs. Depress your shoulder blades. Lift your butt and knees off the floor. Keep your back and hips level (straight). Hold for ten seconds.

Step 2: Do only three reps to start, and focus on maintaining the contraction of the core muscles. It is harder and more effective that way.

Too Difficult? Try fewer reps and a shorter hold. Or don't lift your knees off the floor.

depress shoulder blades

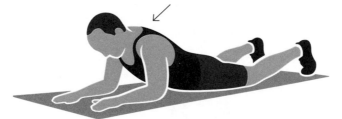

don't let hips sink or back sag

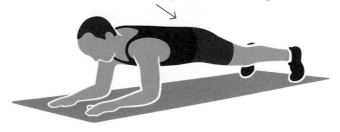

NUMBER 23

Side Plank

Equipment Needed: Foam pad.

Why Bother? This enhances lateral hip and core stability. Worth having, especially if you have knee or low-back problems. It works on the obliques, or side core muscles.

Step 1: Lie on your side, up on one elbow, opposite hand on your hip. Engage your abs and glutes. Lift your hip and knees off the pad. Make sure your body stays in alignment. Hold for ten seconds. Repeat only three times.

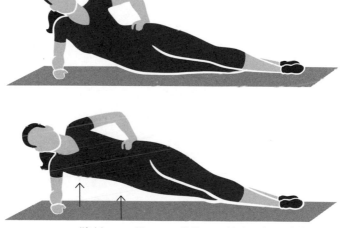

engage core, lift hips and knees off floor, with back straight

Bill Says: *If this is too hard, try the exercise on the floor and with knees bent.*

STRENGTH TRAINING

NUMBER 24

Crunch*

Equipment Needed: Foam pad.

Why Bother? Great for building abs. A shallow sit-up done slowly and with control is just as good as, and much safer than, the old military, full sit-up.

Step 1: Lie on your back with one or both knees bent. Place hands behind the head to support the neck. Contract your abs and use them to lift your shoulders slightly off the floor (about four inches). Don't over-flex your neck. Hold for three to five seconds. Do three sets of ten reps.

Do It Right. Do not lift all the way up. The full power crunches of yesteryear put too much stress on your back.

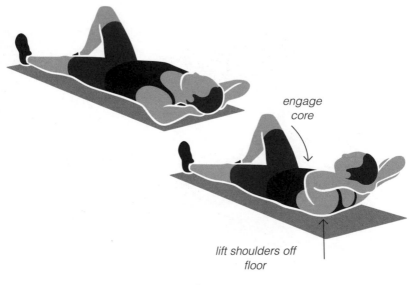

engage
core

lift shoulders off
floor

Bill Says: *Do not do sit-ups with a twist. The twist comes from the lower back, just what you do not want. The safest sit-up is a shallow one, like this.*

NUMBER 25

TRX Rip Trainer "Drag"*

Equipment Needed: We show this with the TRX Rip Trainer, but you could do it as easily with a cable machine (anchored at waist height) or elastic tube.

Why Bother? This looks too easy to bother with but it's not. In fact, it is a nice, stable way to exercise your whole body one last time for the day. It builds endurance and particularly enhances mid- and low-back strength and core stabilization.

Step 1: Stand at a TRX Rip Trainer or a cable machine, facing the anchor point (at midlevel). Hold the Rip Trainer bar in both hands, knees slightly bent and arms straight out, keeping some tension on the bar.

Step 2: Depress your shoulder blades and pull the bar back until it touches your chest. Hold for thirty seconds (up to a minute). Repeat with the cord on the opposite side.

Too Easy? Step back farther and increase the resistance.

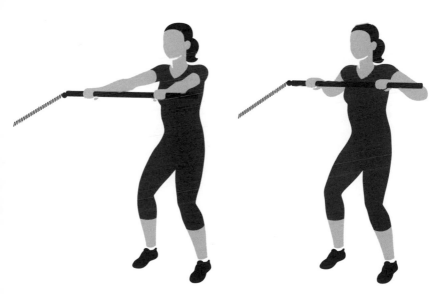

Putting It All Together

Well, that's a lot of weight to throw at you all at once. How do you parse it out and make sure you are getting a good balance in your forty-five-minute workout? Well, when he's training a client, Bill uses a Cheat Sheet, or Day Chart, so he knows the workout contains some of each category of exercise and that the sequence flows and is balanced.

The Day Charts that follow are just an example of a typical balanced strength workout, using different parts of your body. You can choose your exercises; just be sure you pick one or two from each category. Do ten to twelve repetitions. As you adapt, increase weights and do only eight reps. Stay with each of these Day Charts for two to three weeks until you master the movement before moving on.

Chart Day 1

10 minutes of Warm-ups (see Chapter Eight)

Weights:
Two lower body 1) Squats, page 122
                     2) Split Squats, page 123

Two upper body, pulling exercises:
                1) One-Armed Dumbbell Row, page 130
                2) Pull Down (with machine), page 129
Rotation exercise: Rotation/Chop with Medicine Ball, page 136

Combination pattern: Bend, Pull, Overhead Press, page 144, and Squat, Arm Curl, page 143

Specialized exercise: Rotator Cuff External Rotation with Dumbbell, page 148, Side Plank, page 151, and
Hip Extension Lift, page 149

5-minute cool down: Cool down means gentle activity such as
walking followed by stretching key muscles used during exercise,
such as quadriceps or hamstrings.

Chart Day 2

10 minutes of Warm-ups (Chapter Eight)

Weights:
Two lower body 1) The Lunge, page 126, with hands behind head
2) Lateral Lunge, page 128
Two upper body, pushing exercises
1) Chest Press (Bench), page 132
2) Single-Arm Cable Press, page 134

Rotation exercise: Rotation/Chop with Cable Machine, page 138

Combination: Back Step Lunge Row, page 142, with cable (or
whatever combination you didn't do on Day 1)

Specialized exercise: "I's" and "T's" with Dumbbells, page 146,
Plank, page 150, and Crunch, page 152

5-minute cool down: Gentle activity. Include quad stretch after this
workout. Overworking muscles can make us stiff and inflexible if
we don't stretch after working out.

What About Static Stretching?

Often I get this question on the road: Where did stretching go? The short answer, from Bill, is that old-fashioned static stretches—with a thirty- to ninety-second hold, like the good old runner's calf stretch—are not done as much anymore because there are other options. Dynamic stretches, like the ones in our warm-up, are more effective. Watch a ski race today, and you'll see the skier kicking his or her legs vigorously back and forth and from side to side, dramatically. Same for runners: Dynamic stretching is the modern model.

Having said that, static stretches still have a place, especially where a joint or muscle group has gotten disproportionally tight on one side. If you are going to do static stretches, for special situations, it's best to do them after your workout. Or, if you're really stiff in a particular spot, do a static stretch before and after, but integrate it into the relevant dynamic stretches.

The Rhythm of These Sessions

These sessions are designed to have a certain rhythm. Not on Day 1 or even Day 20, when you're still feeling your way. But in time. For example, the warm-ups are intended to build a little, over their course. By the end—certainly by the time of the fast footwork segment—you want to be going for it.

The same pattern is true, in a way, with the strength-building exercises. They're all comparatively hard; they can all have you breathing hard, depending on how you do them. But they, too, are designed to build, over the course of the workout. Begin to work pretty hard when you start with the squats. Be working harder by the time you get to the lunges. Build a little during the later pull-and-push segment. And really go for it in the rotational exercises and, especially, the compound exercises. The latter really lend themselves to a vigorous workout, with more resistance, less rest, and more weight. Go *only* to failure (quit when you aren't doing them right every time)! But over time, you can build to quite the little workout on these babies.

Then taper off as you get into the special-purpose exercises, like the weighted "I's" and "T's," and hip extension lifts, if you do those. Take it down. But toy with that rhythm as you get into all this. It makes it more fun. And it burns a ton of calories while doing all the magic of strength training.

Weekly Plan

How you allocate the days is up to you. But there should be four days of aerobics (two Long and Slow and two Endurance) and two days of strength. Always leave a day between strength-training sessions. Also, be sure to alternate the easy and hard days of aerobics. Each day's workout also includes a ten- to fifteen-minute warm-up and five-minute cool-down.

A basic pattern for the week might look like this:

MONDAY: Strength training

TUESDAY: Aerobics (Long and Slow)

WEDNESDAY: Endurance aerobics or Intervals

THURSDAY: Day off

FRIDAY: Strength training

SATURDAY: Endurance aerobics or Intervals

SUNDAY: Aerobics (Long and Slow) (Harry and I suggest a couple of hours of bike riding or hiking for the joy of it.)

Yearly Plan

A year presents a slightly different problem. It makes sense to have peaks and valleys in your training over the year. Build up for a biking trip—try to "peak" as you head off to the mountains with your bike for a week—or a ski vacation or a week's hike in the mountains. (See "Kedging," page 42.) Take it down some in the weeks or even months that follow—just go on maintenance for a while. Then start a new progression with a new goal to work toward. Got to keep yourself amused.

As Harry said, and as I can personally attest, strength training has more to do with the *quality* of your life than anything else. Your ability to move effectively, your strength, your balance and coordination. And your freedom from pain. All those are radically improved by strength training. We were designed to fall apart as we age, so we are bucking a serious tide here. These exercises are at the heart of it. And they work amazingly well. A guy of sixty or seventy who is in absolutely rotten shape can double the strength in his legs in eight weeks. This stuff works when you are thirty and when you are ninety. Get a great strength-training habit now; maintain it forever.

Nice Going . . . Very Nice Going

Congratulations! You have made it through this sometimes daunting little manual. And we suspect, Harry and I, that if you've come *this* far—dug this deep—you have made a major decision. You have decided to make exercise a serious part of your life. It doesn't *sound* that big—all we're talking about here is working out.

But that's not the way we see it. We think—hell, we *know*—that putting serious exercise at the center of your life is one of the biggest and best things you will ever do. Because the promises we made at the beginning of the book are absolutely true, as you will see, very soon.

Do this stuff and you will enjoy a radical change in energy, fitness, mood, health, optimism, effectiveness, *everything*! Different guy, different girl, by heaven. Seventy percent of aging, out the window and . . . 50 percent of serious illness and accidents gone forever. And you will *feel* entirely different, too. We know because we hear it all the time. I mean *all the time*: "Hey, man, thanks a lot. *It changed my life!*"

We hope you'll stay in touch with us—come to the website, send us an email once in a while, and come back to this little book regularly. But mostly stay in touch with yourself, your *real* self, this time. The great goal in life, I modestly suggest, is "*to live a life fully realized.*" Will exercise alone do all that? Of course not. But it is the rock on which the effort may stand. Try it. You'll see.

About the Authors

Chris Crowley and Henry S. Lodge, M.D., are the co-authors of the *New York Times* bestselling *Younger Next Year* books, which have sold more than a million and a half copies and have been translated into twenty languages worldwide. The *Younger Next Year* books have been called "the best thing ever written" about fitness and wellness for that generation.

Chris Crowley, a former Wall Street litigator (Davis Polk & Wardwell), is also the coauthor, with Tufts professor Jen Sacheck, Ph.D., of *Thinner This Year*, the how-to book on diet and exercise on which this book is significantly based. These days, Chris spends most of his time as a keynote speaker on the revolution in behavior and aging. He also writes about those topics in his fortnightly newsletter, which is available on his website, Youngernextyear. com. He lives with his wife, portraitist Hilary Cooper, in New York City and Lakeville, Connecticut.

Henry S. Lodge, M.D., FACP, is the Robert Burch Family Professor of Medicine at the Columbia University Medical Center. He is recognized in *Who's Who, Who's Who in Medicine and*

Health Care, and *Who's Who in Science and Engineering.* He is consistently listed as "one of the best doctors," in surveys such as "Best Doctors in New York," "America," and "Best Doctors in the World." He is a practicing, board-certified internist, and heads a twenty-doctor academic group practice in Manhattan, where he lives.

Bill Fabrocini, P.T., C.S.C.S., is a clinical specialist in orthopedic physical therapy and a sports performance training coach. During his twenty-five-year career, he has designed exercise programs for companies such as Massachusetts General Hospital and Aspen Ski Company. He has trained a lot of famous athletes, including N.B.A. M.V.P. David Robinson, Olympic medalists Chris Klug and Gretchen Bleiler, and tennis grand slam champion Martina Navratilova. Bill also created the strength-training program in *Thinner This Year* and in this book. His two DVDs that supplement the exercise portion in this book are "Preparation for Movement" and "The Sacred 25 and Beyond," which are available at youngernextyear.com.

Riggs Klika, Ph.D., is currently a visiting professor of sports medicine at Pepperdine University in Malibu, California. During his long career, he has focused on aerobic exercise. A former team physiologist for the US Ski Team, he has been a trainer of professional athletes all his life. One of his recent ventures was establishing a serious exercise program for cancer survivors, in which he had amazing success with his clients. He created the aerobic exercise portion in *Thinner This Year* and this book.

Acknowledgments

D eep thanks first to Bill Fabrocini, who really is the brains and spirit of much of this book. I spent *years* with him, learning this stuff for *Thinner This Year* and doing this book. He is simply the best in the field. And thanks, too, to Riggs Klika, with whom I have spent so much good time and from whom I have learned so much.

And, of course, to Harry: One simply could not have a better, wiser, or steadier coauthor and friend. He is the brains of the whole *Younger Next Year* enterprise.

Very special thanks to Ruth Sullivan, who pulled this together in the first place and put up with my passionate views on exercise, language, and everything else (apparently not a restful experience). She brought extraordinary experience, energy, and intelligence to the project, from first to last. When she is done, it looks easy. It is not.

And to our beloved Suzie Bolotin, the Wise Minerva whose idea this was and who oversaw it from afar, kept us all from going crazy, and made it all happen. We are blessed to have her.

Finally, to my wife, Hilary Cooper, who has read every word of this fifty times and still manages to care and counsel.

Index

OVER 1 MILLION COPIES SOLD

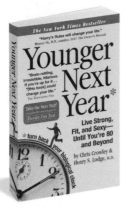

Dr. Henry Lodge provides the science. Chris Crowley provides the motivation. And through their *New York Times* bestselling program, you'll discover how to put off 70 percent of the normal problems of aging—weakness, sore joints, bad balance—and eliminate 50 percent of serious illness and injury. How, in fact, to become functionally younger every year for the next five to ten years, and continue to live with newfound vitality and pleasure.

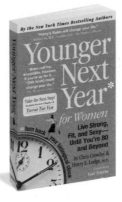

A book of hope, *Younger Next Year for Women* shows how to live brilliantly for the three decades or more after menopause. The key is found in Harry's Rules, a program of exercise, diet, and maintaining emotional connections that will be natural for you, as a woman, to implement. With a foreword by Gail Sheehy.

"I loved the book! It's got all the tools that women need to achieve longer, sexier, and more passionate lives."

—Hilda Hutcherson, M.D., Clinical Professor of Obstetrics and Gynecology, and Director of the Center for Sexual Health, Columbia University

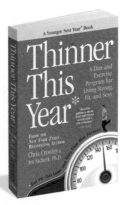

Here's the how-to book for the new revolution in aging. It's about how you move, with exercises that will be the greatest driver of positive change in your body. About how you eat, from avoiding foods with solid fats and added sugars to skipping the supplements. And the payoff is amazing: newfound energy, strength, optimism, health, and weight loss.

"Chock-full of easy recipes, meal plans, and exercise diagrams."
—*The Wall Street Journal*

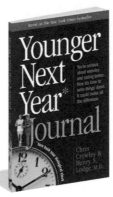

Is it a cardio day or a strength day? What's your resting heart rate? A 52-week, prompted fill-in organizer and date book that makes it easy to record what you're doing, and when, *The Younger Next Year Journal* is an essential tool for living the program day to day.

Available Wherever Books Are Sold

workman.com